Contents

Preface

This book represents the consolidation of a number of activities undertaken by WHO in recent years to review the available evidence on tobacco use by women and to identify the most promising strategies for tobacco control.

The events leading to the publication of this book began on 31 May 1989, the second World No-Tobacco Day, when a round-table meeting on "women and tobacco" was held at WHO headquarters in Geneva. It was subsequently agreed that the proceedings of this meeting should be edited and a paper produced on the subject. In the course of the preparation of this paper, it became clear that the subject deserved more extensive consideration. Accordingly, information on women and tobacco was gathered from a variety of countries and a draft monograph was produced. The monograph was reviewed by a group of experts who met in Geneva from 10 to 14 June 1991, following which it was revised.

This book is intended to inform all those concerned with this previously under-researched and under-publicized subject. It is primarily aimed at decision-makers and, in particular, at the staff of ministries of health, education, labour and social welfare, legislators, nongovernmental organizations and community leaders. It is also expected that this monograph will prompt the opening of new avenues of research and the more systematic documentation of issues relating to women and tobacco.

Author and editorial advisers

Author

Dr Claire Chollat-Traquet joined the World Health Organization in 1974; at present she is a scientist with the WHO Programme on Tobacco or Health.

Editorial advisers

Leading experts on tobacco control have provided information and acted as advisers for this book. Their contribution is gratefully acknowledged.

Dr Michele Bloch is a manager of women's programmes at the Advocacy Institute in Washington, DC, USA and was formerly Director of the Women vs. Smoking Network in the United States.

Dr Dulce Estrelle-Gust is a community psychiatrist, currently working in the Philippines on psychosocial factors related to the working environment.

Dr Lorraine Greaves is a professor of sociology at Fanshawe College of Applied Arts and Technology in London, Canada.

Dr Alan Lopez is an epidemiologist with the WHO Programme on Tobacco or Health; prior to joining the programme, he worked for over a decade in the Division of Epidemiological Surveillance and Health Situation and Trend Assessment, World Health Organization.

Dr Judith Mackay is director of the Asian Consultancy on Tobacco Control in Hong Kong; she is currently a member of the WHO Expert Advisory Panel on Tobacco or Health.

Dr Keith Rothwell is a scientist; during recent years he has been a consultant with the WHO Programme on Tobacco or Health.

ix

Dr Annie J. Sasco is a medical epidemiologist in the French National Institute of Health and Medical Research (INSERM), Paris, France; she is currently on secondment to the Unit of Analytical Epidemiology at the International Agency for Research on Cancer, Lyon, France.

Dr Elena Stroot is a researcher at the Institute of Prevention of Noncommunicable Diseases in Moscow, Russian Federation.

Acknowledgements

The author wishes to acknowledge the contributions of the following WHO staff members in reviewing the monograph:

Dr M. A. Belsey, Programme Manager, Maternal and Child Health and Family Planning, Division of Family Health, Geneva, Switzerland; Ms B. J. Ferguson, Technical Officer, Adolescent Health, Division of Family Health, Geneva, Switzerland; Dr I. Gyárfás, Chief Medical Officer, Cardiovascular Diseases, Division of Noncommunicable Diseases and Health Technology, Geneva, Switzerland; Dr V. Koroltchouk, Scientist, Cancer and Palliative Care, Division of Noncommunicable Diseases and Health Technology, Geneva, Switzerland; Dr J. R. Menchaca, Programme Manager, Tobacco or Health, Division of Health Protection and Promotion, Geneva, Switzerland; Dr P. Nordet, Medical Officer, Cardiovascular Diseases, Division of Noncommunicable Diseases and Health Technology, Geneva, Switzerland; Dr T. Piha, Community Health Specialist, Regional Adviser on Tobacco or Health, WHO Regional Office for Europe, Copenhagen, Denmark; Dr A. Pio, Programme Manager, Control of Acute Respiratory Infections, Division of Diarrhoeal and Acute Respiratory Disease Control, Geneva, Switzerland; Dr H. Restrepo, Coordinator, Health Promotion, WHO Regional Office for the Americas / Pan American Sanitary Bureau, Washington, DC, USA.

The author would also like to acknowledge the contributions of Dr A. Amos, Lecturer in Health Education and Director of the MSc programme on Health Promotion and Health Education, at the University of Edinburgh, Edinburgh, Scotland, in assisting in the final editing of this book, and of Mrs M. Villanueva in undertaking the literary research for the monograph.

Thanks are also due to the nongovernmental organizations dealing with the issue of women and tobacco which kindly offered information, as well as the many others who contributed to the production of the monograph. The preparation of this monograph was supported in part by the Japan Shipbuilding Industry Foundation, whose assistance is gratefully acknowledged.

Chapter 1

Women and tobacco: the issues at stake

Women smokers are numbered in millions throughout the world, and several million more are dependent on tobacco used in other ways. The number of women smokers increases daily, not only because of the world's fast-growing population, but also because smoking cigarettes is being fostered and encouraged worldwide for commercial gain and, in spite of incontrovertible evidence on the toll of death, disease, and disability that is being caused, many governments have remained ambivalent towards a problem that has implications for excise and tax revenue, health and welfare expenditure, and political expediency.

The incidence of smoking-related diseases and concomitant death rates have increased rapidly among women in many developed countries in recent years. In most countries, there are no epidemiological indications of a likely decrease in the near future and the continuing uptake of smoking in these countries gives cause to expect a continuing increase in both disease incidence and death rates. In most developing countries, cigarette smoking, so far maintained at a low level, is being fiercely promoted by the tobacco companies. As more women become dependent on tobacco, the effect will be an inexorable toll on health and well-being; and the impact will be such as to prevent the achievement of WHO's goal of health for all by the year 2000.

Tobacco use can be compared to an epidemic; it spreads within societies and from one society, and one population, to another. There follows in its wake an epidemic of smoking-related disease, albeit after a lapse in time. In the absence of tobacco, some diseases such as lung cancer might be almost nonexistent in women, and others such as ischaemic heart disease and chronic lung disease would be rarer.

Until recently, the incidence and mortality rates from smoking-related diseases had been much lower among women than among men and suppositions that women may be more resistant to tobacco have arisen. It is now clear, however, that women are not only susceptible to the same tobacco-related diseases as men, but are also affected by other specific conditions.

In the developed countries, where smoking by women is well established, the challenge is twofold: to halt the rapid escalation in tobacco dependence that is currently occurring in many areas and to register more success in reducing the prevalence and intensity of smoking by women.

There are many areas of the world, particularly in the developing countries, where tobacco use is still at a low level and may as yet even be nonexistent among women. Here is where future disease could be effectively prevented. There is, however, a lack of knowledge on tobacco use by women in most countries and efforts to obtain more factual information are needed so that countermeasures can be developed and used more effectively.

While there is a need for further information, there is sufficient evidence for public health action on tobacco use by women not to be delayed. This monograph is thus intended to provide background information on a wide range of aspects of smoking by women and to identify the strategies available to combat the growing problem of tobacco use among women.

Chapter 2

Women and tobacco use: patterns and trends

Tobacco is the single largest cause of premature adult death throughout the world. Over the next 30 years tobacco-related deaths among women will more than double, so that by the year 2020 well over a million adult women will die every year from tobacco-related illnesses. Currently, in the developed world, the prevalence of smoking among women is approximately 20–35%, whereas in the developing world, it is estimated at 2–10%.

In the developed countries, smoking by women was socially unacceptable for many years. However, by the mid-20th century, in most developed countries, smoking by women had increased rapidly. As the health hazards of tobacco became apparent, the prevalence of smoking among men declined in some developed countries. Prevalence rates among women did not begin to decline until later and then only in a few countries; the two rates are currently converging in several countries. Today, in many developed countries, smoking is predominantly a practice of young women, women with limited education, and women of low socioeconomic status.

In the past, cultural norms were a powerful deterrent to women's smoking in the developing world, although there have always been areas in which women have practised traditional forms of tobacco use. Currently, in the developing world, smoking is linked with a cosmopolitan and affluent life-style. With increasing urbanization and career-oriented education, and increasing spending power, many young women who aspire to this life-style have taken up smoking. There is grave concern that these aspirations, fuelled by aggressive tobacco marketing, will result in increased prevalence rates among women in developing countries, further compounding their present difficulties.

This chapter provides the statistical evidence for urging strong tobacco control efforts in both the developed and developing world to decrease the epidemic of tobacco use among women. While there is already enough evidence to justify urgent action, knowledge of the overall situation among women in developing countries is hampered by cultural reticence to admitting to tobacco use and by the scarcity of survey data. To complement tobacco control interventions more effectively and to monitor future trends, continuous surveillance will be needed.

Tobacco (*Nicotiana*, a member of the Solanaceae family) is a native plant of the Americas, where it was used for ceremonial and medicinal purposes for thousands of years by many of the indigenous populations. It is believed that the practice of smoking was also known in Asia long before Columbus visited the New World. Tobacco was one of many plants brought from North America to Europe in the 1500s by the early European explorers and the use of tobacco quickly spread through the European populations. Tobacco was also introduced to other continents as early as the 1600s by explorers and missionaries. In Europe, Portuguese men were the first users of tobacco (usually smoked in pipes), but European women also used tobacco, both in pipes and as snuff. During this period, arguments for sexual equality were already being made to gain permission and social acceptability for women's smoking.

The advent of machine-manufactured cigarettes in the late 1800s was a major factor in cigarettes becoming the dominant form of tobacco use in the early twentieth century. Colonization in many parts of the world brought about dramatic changes in agricultural patterns; colonized countries were encouraged to grow tobacco, and they continued to do so after independence because of the substantial earnings from tobacco exports, making it the most widely grown commercial non-food plant in the world. Through exploration, advertising, marketing, and widespread tobacco cultivation, cigarette use continued to spread throughout the world, and progressively became superimposed upon traditional tobacco uses.

Smoking has not always been socially acceptable for men and it has been even less so for women. In 1606, two University Decrees were issued by Cambridge University which prohibited any student or other member of the University from drinking excessively or using tobacco. During the 1800s and early 1900s, tobacco use by women and children was largely unacceptable. In most developed countries, smoking by women was considered to be vulgar, improper and even immoral, and the anti-smoking movements in several countries were often led by women or women's organizations. Opponents of tobacco believed that it exploited the poor and was immoral, unhealthy, hazardous and unfeminine; however, such attitudes began to change with the coming of women's emancipation, combined not only with their increasing employment in paid occupations but also their development of careers of their own and a decreasing dependence on men for their livelihood.

During the First World War, sending cigarettes to soldiers was deemed patriotic, which effectively put an end to the organized anti-smoking movement. As women became more emancipated in North America and Europe, through suffrage and dress reform, smoking became increasingly acceptable.

4

In the 1920s, women started smoking in public as a sign of emancipation and equality, although they smoked considerably fewer cigarettes than men (2.4 versus 7.2 cigarettes per day on average in the United States in 1929). Smoking became fashionable in the 1930s, particularly among women in the cities; in the United States, 18.1% of women and 52.5% of men were smokers by 1935.

During the Second World War, as women contributed to the national war effort, smoking by women became associated with going out to work, and with independence, emancipation and patriotism. Women were not only working like men, but adopting their behaviour as well. After the war, the prevalence of smoking among women was about 40% in the United Kingdom, 30% in Australia and 25% in the United States.

- In the United Kingdom, by 1950 the prevalence of smoking was 38% for women and 62% for men. Prevalence rates among women reached 45% in 1966 before starting to fall as the risks of smoking became evident (*1*).

Although some studies had been carried out in 1939 and in the 1940s (mainly in Germany and the Netherlands), there was little scientific evidence on the harmful effects of tobacco use until the 1940s. In 1950, it began to be recognized that cigarette smoking was associated with serious disease risks. A number of studies carried out in the United Kingdom and the United States showed an association between smoking and certain forms of cancer, particularly lung cancer.

Nevertheless, cigarette sales continued to increase throughout the developed world until the mid-1970s, when information campaigns against tobacco began to take effect. During the 1970s and 1980s, stagnation in the growth of the global tobacco economy due to reduced demand became evident. As profits are threatened, the tobacco industry has started massive marketing in the developing countries. Long-term expansion will be seen in developing countries because of their dependence on the substantial export earnings from tobacco and revenue from domestic use. Moreover, the public health campaigns about the hazards of tobacco use are at an early stage in many developing countries.

In some countries, the change from traditional forms of tobacco use can be seen as recently as during the last 20 years. In Bangladesh the majority of smokers used hookah in the 1970s, while the recent smokers are beginning to take up bidi smoking.

5

Global overview

Tobacco use

The foremost way in which tobacco is used throughout the world is for smoking in cigarettes, but in some developing countries, although cigarette use has increased since the 1940s, other traditional uses continue to predominate, particularly among rural and isolated communities.

Tobacco use can be classified under six principal headings: as cigarettes, bidis, cigars, pipe tobacco, snuff and for chewing. There are variants of usage within each group. Thus, for example, in addition to manufactured ("white") cigarettes, kreteks (cigarettes containing tobacco and cloves) are smoked in Indonesia, and papyrosi (cigarettes in which the conventional tip is replaced by a long paper tube) are smoked in many parts of the USSR.

The tobacco in manufactured cigarettes is cut in very thin strands, approximately 1 mm in diameter, and a form of "fine cut" tobacco is sold loose for smokers to roll their own cigarettes. Hand-rolled cigarettes usually yield more tar and nicotine, because the tobacco is stronger and the paper used is also thicker and less permeable than the wrapper of manufactured cigarettes; on the other hand, they often contain less tobacco than manufactured cigarettes.

The bidi (beedi, biri) is common throughout south-east Asia and consists of tobacco flakes or powder, loosely packed and rolled in a dried tendu or temburni leaf. The dhumti in India is similar, but the tobacco is rolled in a leaf of the jackfruit tree. Other bidi-like smoking devices may have banana leaves or even newspaper as the wrapper.

Cigars are made from cured tobacco leaves rolled and wrapped in a dried tobacco leaf and are produced in a variety of shapes and sizes. They are also known by different names in different localities: e.g. the cheroot and chutta in India; and khi yo, ya muan and tra kai in regions of Thailand. All these traditional smoking devices tend to use oriental or native varieties of tobacco and the smoke is invariably extremely strong, containing high levels of tar, nicotine and carbon monoxide.

Pipe smoking, probably the oldest recorded form of smoking, is practised in almost all countries and the shapes and names for pipes are legion. However, one variety of pipe common to almost all countries in the Eastern Mediterranean and parts of Asia is the water pipe (hookah, goza or hubble-bubble), a device in which the smoke bubbles through water before being inhaled. The hookah apparatus also has many shapes, sizes and names in different countries or areas in which it is common. Hookah tobacco shows regional variations;

6

it may contain only cured tobacco leaves or the tobacco may have been fermented in molasses, honey or fruit juices. The smoke again tends to be strong but is rendered less harsh by being bubbled through the water; however, it has a high carbon monoxide content because the tobacco is ignited and kept alight by covering it with pieces of glowing charcoal. In some Eastern Mediterranean countries, hookah smoking by women is often a social event.

Snuff is used in two different forms: as dried, finely powdered tobacco which is inhaled through the nostrils or as moist, coarsely ground tobacco which is retained in various parts of the mouth.

When tobacco is chewed, it is usually mixed with other materials. For example, pan masala ("pan") is extremely common in India where it is used by at least 20 million people, and may contain some of the following substances: tobacco, betel nut, dried dates, catechu, slaked lime, menthol and spices such as cardamom, clove, mace and cinnamon. Obviously the mixture can vary and tobacco does not always have to be one of the ingredients. Throughout south-east Asia and in many North African and Eastern Mediterranean countries, tobacco is chewed in combination with flavourings, frequently lime, and has many names: gazare (Afghanistan and Pakistan), mainpuri and naswar (Pakistan), makla (Algeria), alshammah (Saudi Arabia), shammah (Yemen), khaini (India and Nepal), nachouk (Egypt) and zarda, which is used in Nepal and includes perfumes and spices and in its more expensive forms, musk.

Mishri (masheri) is a form of burnt tobacco which is used for cleaning teeth and is often retained in the mouth. In many developing countries where smoking by women is often socially unacceptable, tobacco chewing seems to be more acceptable and is relatively widespread. Reverse smoking, where a chutta, dhumti or bidi is smoked with the lighted end in the mouth is often more common among women in areas where their smoking is acceptable.

Tobacco-related morbidity and mortality

Currently, tobacco use is estimated to account for 3 million deaths per year, about half a million of which are among women, reflecting their previous patterns of tobacco consumption. Slightly more than half of these deaths occur in the developed world, where smoking has been at a higher level and over a longer period than in the developing world. Over the past decade or so, there have been significant changes in consumption patterns, with consumption and smoking prevalence rising in many developing coun-

7

tries, especially among men, but remaining unchanged or even falling considerably in some developed countries, most notably the United Kingdom and the United States.

- In China, for example, which accounts for almost one-third of the entire population of the developing world, the consumption of cigarettes increased from 500 thousand million in 1978 to 1400 thousand million in 1987. This represents one-quarter of the world's total cigarette consumption; in 1990, this proportion had risen to about 30%. About 61% of Chinese men smoke, compared with slightly less than 7% of women over 15 years of age (2).

Surveys conducted during the 1980s indicated that in almost 60% of developing countries, fewer than 10% of women were smokers, compared with about 30% of women in most developed countries. Among women, death rates from lung cancer, a very reliable marker of the evolution of the cigarette smoking epidemic, are rising virtually throughout the developed world and consequently the full effects of the massive adoption of cigarette smoking by women after the Second World War are yet to be seen.

In many developing countries, low life expectancy has masked the onset of the chronic smoking-related diseases. However, as life expectancy in these countries improves, the effects of the continuing adoption of smoking by women will become more evident. In Brazil, for example, it is projected that life expectancy will reach about 68 years of age by the year 2000; however, it is likely to remain considerably lower in Africa for the foreseeable future. Nevertheless, a decisive factor affecting the mortality from smoking-related diseases will be the rates at which women take up smoking in these countries, which is influenced by factors such as traditions, social and cultural norms, beliefs, income and the targeting of women by the tobacco industry through advertising.

In view of these trends, what will be the likely future health effects of previous tobacco consumption, particularly smoking? At the global level, the annual number of tobacco-related deaths is expected to rise dramatically from 3 million to about 10 million by the year 2020; many of these deaths will be among women. Only if there were to be a substantial fall in smoking prevalence among adolescents would this epidemic of tobacco-related deaths be moderated, since the majority of these deaths will occur among the youth and young adults of today, born between about 1950 and 1980, precisely the period when cigarette smoking was adopted extensively on a worldwide scale. Conversely, the majority of the tobacco-related deaths which occur today are among smokers born before 1950. Of the projected 10 million tobacco-related deaths in the year 2020, about 3 million are expected to occur in China alone on the basis of current smoking patterns. However, if the prevalence of smoking among women increases in developing countries, future projections will need to be revised upwards.

Worldwide prevalence of tobacco consumption by women

While the extent of the epidemic of tobacco-related deaths can be deduced for developed countries where vital statistics and data on the prevalence of smoking are readily available, precise prevalence data for tobacco use in individual developing countries are less readily available, especially the prevalence of smoking among women. Assessing the epidemic is thus more difficult. The best available data, presented in Tables 1–6, give an indication

Table 1. Prevalence of cigarette smoking among women in the Region of the Americas*

Country	Prevalence (%)	Date of survey	Source
Argentina	27 (38)†	1988	(a)
Bahamas	4	1989	(b)
Bolivia	38	1986	(c)
Brazil	33 (30 – 33)†	1990 (1986)	National survey
Canada	25.8	1986	(b)
Chile	31 (58)†	1988	(a)
Colombia	18 (21)†	1988	(a) (d)
Costa Rica	20 (12.4)†	1988 (1986)	(a) (d)
Cuba	25.5	1988	(e)
Dominican Republic	13.6	1989	(e)
Ecuador	16 (8)†	1988	(a) (d)
El Salvador	12	1988	(a) (d)
Guatemala (urban areas)	17.7 (4)†	1989 (1987)	(e)
Guyana	4	—	(e)
Honduras	11	1988	(a) (d)
Jamaica	27 (6.2)†	1988 (1989)	(d)
Mexico	17	1988	(d)
Panama	20	1983	(e)
Paraguay	(7)†	NA	NA
Peru	17	1988	(a) (c) (d)
Trinidad and Tobago	5	1986–89	NA
United States of America	26	1990	(e)
Uruguay	23 (44)†	1988	(a)
Venezuela	23 (34)†	1988	(a) (d)

* No data are available for Antigua and Barbuda, Barbados, Belize, Dominica, Grenada, Haiti, Nicaragua, Saint Kitts and Nevis, Saint Lucia, Saint Vincent and the Grenadines, and Suriname.
† Data refer to women of childbearing age.
(a) Gallup, 1988.
(b) National health department.
(c) American Cancer Society.
(d) WHO/PAHO: CD33/24, Rev. 1 (unpublished document; available from WHO Regional Office for the Americas, Washington, DC 20037, USA).
(e) Indicative figures collected by WHO from various sources.

9

Table 2. Prevalence of cigarette smoking among women in the European Region*

Country	Prevalence (%)	Date of survey	Source
Austria	28	1984	(a)
Belgium	28	1988	(b)
Bulgaria	17	1989	(a)
Czechoslovakia	28	1990	(c)
Denmark	45	1988	(b)
Finland	20	1988	(a)
France	30	1991	(a)
Germany	27	1988	(b)
Greece	26	1988	(b)
Hungary	23	1986	(a)
Iceland	32	1990	(d)
Ireland	31	1988	(b)
Israel	25	1988	(a)
Italy	26	1988	(b)
Luxembourg	30	1988	(b)
Malta	22	1991	(c)
Netherlands	37	1988	(b)
Norway	34	1990–91	(a)
Poland	35	1989	NA
Portugal	12	1988	(b)
Spain	28	1988	(b)
Sweden	26	1986–89	(d)
Switzerland	28	1989	(a)
USSR (Moscow)	10†	1986	NA
United Kingdom of Great Britain and Northern Ireland	32	1988	(b)
Yugoslavia	36†	NA	(c)

* No data are available for Albania, Belarus, Monaco, Romania, San Marino and Turkey.
† Data refer to a limited area.
(a) Communication from Member States.
(b) Europe Against Cancer.
(c) Countrywide Integrated Noncommunicable Diseases Intervention programme (CINDI).
(d) Indicative figures collected by WHO from various sources.

Table 3. Prevalence of cigarette smoking among women in the African Region*

Country	Prevalence (%)	Date of survey	Source
Côte d'Ivoire	1	1981	(a)
Ghana	1–6	NA	(a)
Guinea	1	1981	(a)
Mauritius	7	1986–89	(a) (b)
Nigeria	10	1990	(c)
Swaziland	7	1989	(a)
Zambia	4–7	1984	(a) (b)

* No data are available for Algeria, Angola, Benin, Botswana, Burkina Faso, Burundi, Cameroon, Cape Verdi, Central African Republic, Chad, Comoros, Congo, Equatorial Guinea, Ethiopia, Gabon, Gambia, Guinea-Bissau, Kenya, Lesotho, Liberia, Madagascar, Malawi, Mali, Mauritania, Mozambique, Namibia, Niger, Rwanda, Sao Tome and Principe, Senegal, Seychelles, Sierra Leone, South Africa, Togo, Uganda, United Republic of Tanzania, Zaire and Zimbabwe.
(a) Indicative figures collected by WHO from various sources.
(b) Reference 3.
(c) *Tobacco and society in Nigeria: research trends in production, promotion and consumption of cigarettes.* Paper presented at the 7th World Conference on Tobacco and Health, Perth 1990.

Table 4. Prevalence of cigarette smoking among women in the Eastern Mediterranean Region*

Country	Prevalence (%)	Date of survey	Source
Bahrain	20	1985	(a)
Cyprus	8	1991	(a)
Egypt	2	1981	(a)
Iraq	5	1990	(a)
Jordan	18 students	1989	(b)
Kuwait	12	NA	(a)
Lebanon	39 students	1975	(a)
Morocco	9.1–14.9	NA	(c)
Oman	3–9	1990	(a)
Pakistan	6 (39 users)	1982	(a)
Qatar	3–9	1990	(a)
Sudan	19	1986	NA
Tunisia	6	1984	(a)
United Arab Emirates	3–9	1990	(a)

    * No data are available for Afghanistan, Djibouti, Islamic Republic of Iran, Libyan Arab Jamahiriya, Saudi Arabia, Somalia, Syrian Arab Republic and Yemen.
    (a) Indicative figures collected by WHO from various sources.
    (b) *Jordan times*, 30 May 1989.
    (c) The prevalence of smoking among women in Morocco was given as 14.9% in reference *4*; however, information received by WHO from the Ministry of Health, 26 March 1990, indicated that the prevalence was 9.1%.

Table 5. Prevalence of cigarette smoking among women in the South-East Asia Region*

Country	Prevalence (%)	Date of survey	Source
Bangladesh	20 (1)†	1984 (1982)†	(a) (c) (d)
India	3‡	1984	(c)
Indonesia	10 (3.6)	1990 (1986)	(b) (e)
Mongolia	7	1991	(a)
Myanmar	29†	1989	(b)
Nepal	58	1991	(a)
Sri Lanka	1–3.3§	1989	(f)
Thailand	4	1988	(g)

    * No data are available for Bhutan, Democratic People's Republic of Korea and Maldives.
    † Data refer to women in rural areas and women in two poor village populations, respectively.
    ‡ Data refer to smokers in a rural community. Use of tobacco by women in India may vary from 0% to 67%, depending on the area chosen and the form of tobacco use surveyed.
    § Data refer to a survey of 1% of towns, 3.3% of suburbs and 1% of villages in Sri Lanka.
    (a) Indicative figures collected by WHO from various sources.
    (b) Reference *3*.
    (c) *Smoking and Health*. Report of a WHO Regional Seminar.
    (d) Cohen N. Smoking and survival prospects in Bangladesh. *World health forum*, 1982, 3: 441 – 444.
    (e) In: Durston B, Jamrozik K, ed. *The global war. Abstracts of the 7th World Conference on Tobacco and Health, Perth, 1 – 5 April 1990*. Perth, Health Department of Western Australia, 1990, p. 241. Results of household surveys conducted in 1980 and 1986 are given as 3.1% and 3.6%, respectively.
    (f) *Smoking patterns in Sri Lanka 1989*. National Cancer Control Programme, Sri Lanka.
    (g) *Health and Welfare survey on tobacco use, 1988*. Updated in March 1990 by H. Chitanondh, National Committee for Control of Tobacco Use, Ministry of Public Health, Thailand.

Table 6. Prevalence of cigarette smoking among women in the Western Pacific Region*

Country	Prevalence (%)	Date of survey	Source
Australia	27	1986–89	(a)
Brunei Darussalam	7	1980	(b)
Cambodia	—†	1990	(b)
China	8.28 (7.04)‡	1984	(c)
Cook Islands	19	1978	(d)
Fiji (Melanesian)	44§	1980	(d)
Fiji (Indian)	13**	1980	(d)
Japan	14.3 (12.7)	1990 (1989)	(b)
Kiribati	—† †	—	(d)
Malaysia	5	1990	(e)
New Zealand	26	1986–89	(b)
Papua New Guinea	80‡ ‡	1990	(e)
Philippines	18.7 (21.9)	1988 (1990)	(f) (e)
Republic of Korea	6.8	1990	(g) (f)
Samoa	22§ §	1978	(d)
Singapore	2.4	1988	(b)
Solomon Islands	10 (33)	1989 (1990)	(f) (e)
Tonga	8	1990	(e)
Vanuatu	10	1990	(e)
Viet Nam	0.3–3.4	1990	(e)

* No data are available for Federated States of Micronesia, Lao People's Democratic Republic, Marshall Islands and Tokelau.

† Prevalence rates among urban and rural populations were 3% and 10%, respectively.

‡ Data refer to prevalence among women over 20 years of age. Figure in parentheses refers to prevalence among women over 15 years of age.

§ Prevalence rates among urban and rural populations were 33% and 50%, respectively.

** Prevalence rates among urban and rural populations were 4% and 22%, respectively.

† † Prevalence rates among urban and rural populations were 74% and 66%, respectively.

‡ ‡ Data refer to a small study of women in certain rural areas.

§ § Prevalence rates among urban and rural populations were 17% and 27%, respectively.

(a) Hill DJ, White VM, Gray NJ. Australian patterns of tobacco smoking in 1989. *Medical journal of Australia,* 1991, 154: 797–801.

(b) Indicative figures collected by WHO from various sources.

(c) Reference 2.

(d) Reference 5.

(e) Regional Working Group on Tobacco or Health, Australia, March 1990.

(f) WHO Regional Office for the Western Pacific. Report of Regional Working Group on Tobacco or Health, Perth 1990.

(g) Hae Sook Lee, Il Soon Kim. Cigarette smoking rates for Koreans for the past 80 years – birth cohort analysis. In: Durston B, Jamrozik K, ed. *The global war. Abstracts of the 7th World Conference on Tobacco and Health, Perth, 1–5 April 1990.* Perth, Health Department of Western Australia, 1990, p. 163.

of the prevalence of smoking among women in the various WHO Member States; however, the quality of the data is variable and the figures should be taken only as a general illustration of comments in the following chapters.

Developed countries

The current situation

In developed countries, the prevalence and intensity of smoking among women show marked variations, depending on factors such as the duration of smoking, the age at which smoking starts, socioeconomic background, educational attainment and nature of occupation. These factors are discussed in Chapter 4. In general, the countries in which smoking was first taken up were the first to show a decline in the prevalence of smoking among women. It should be noted that even in some European countries, such as Greece and Spain, the prevalence of smoking among women appears still to be increasing.

Currently, in some developed countries, the numbers of men and women who smoke are converging, albeit at different rates (Table 7), but with fewer men than women taking up smoking, even this equalization may be destroyed and more women than men may become dependent on tobacco.

- In Australia and the United States, men and women are quitting smoking at about the same rate but more young women than young men are taking up smoking; as a result, the gap between male and female smoking prevalence rates has closed (6, 7). It has been predicted (8), on the basis of current trends in the United States, that there will be more female smokers than male smokers by 1996.
- In Canada, 3.2 million women and 3.3 million men were smokers in 1989 (9).

In addition, there are many other developed countries where the prevalence of smoking among women is not declining as rapidly as it is among men, thus there may also be more female smokers than male smokers in the future. For example, Table 7 suggests that there has been a significant decline in the prevalence of smoking among women in Canada and the United Kingdom and a stabilization or even a very slight decrease in Australia and the United States of America. The data for Finland suggest a slight increase in prevalence among women in the late 1980s.

Prevalence data do not give the total picture, since the ways in which women smoke will also influence the effects tobacco will have on their health. In general, women smoke fewer cigarettes than men and these tend to be lower in tar and nicotine; their patterns of inhalation may also be different. They rarely smoke pipes or large cigars and the use of small cigars tends to be restricted to women in a few social groups and even then only on a few social occasions. Unlike the situation prevailing in many developing

13

Table 7. Prevalence of cigarette smoking in five developed countries

Country	Year							
Australia [a]	1945	1964	1969	1976	1980	1986	1989	
Men (%)	72	58	45	40	40	32	30	
Women (%)	26	28	28	31	31	29	27	
Canada [b]	1965	1970	1975	1981	1983	1985	1989	
Men (%)	61	65	51	44	41	36	33	
Women (%)	38	38	38	35	34	32	30	
Finland	1965	1970	1975	1980	1985	1989		
Men (%)	57	44	40	37	35	34		
Women (%)	14	16	17	16	17	20		
United Kingdom [a]	1956[c]	1961[c]	1965[c]	1972	1976	1980	1984	1988
Men (%)	75	72	68	52	46	42	36	33
Women (%)	42	44	43	41	38	36	32	30
United States of America [d]	1955	1965	1970	1976	1980	1983	1987	1988
Men (%)	53	50	44	42	38	35	32	31
Women (%)	25	32	31	31	29	29	27	26

[a] Data refer to prevalence of daily smoking at 16 years of age and above.
[b] Data refer to prevalence of smoking at 15 years of age and above.
[c] Includes all forms of smoking.
[d] Data refer to prevalence of regular smoking (see Annex 1).
Source : WHO Country Database.

countries, particularly among rural populations, tobacco chewing is rare among women in developed countries.

The situation in eastern Europe and Japan is different from that in other developed countries. In Japan the proportion of women who smoked increased to about 15% during the early 1980s; it has since fallen slightly, but is still high compared with other Asian countries. The low prevalence of smoking among Japanese women relative to women in other developed countries is probably due to the unavailability of cigarettes immediately following the Second World War, combined with traditional attitudes against women smoking. However, current estimates suggest that 12% of girls aged 13–15 years and 26% of girls aged 16–18 years smoke, and health authorities in Japan state that those who leave school early smoke much more. If these higher smoking rates among teenagers persist into adulthood, women in Japan will face appalling health consequences in the future.

There are considerable variations in the patterns of tobacco use in the countries of central and eastern Europe. In some countries, such as Czechoslovakia, Hungary and Poland, smoking follows a pattern similar to that in other developed countries, especially among the urban population; however, in rural areas of these countries, as well as in Bulgaria, Romania and large parts of the former USSR, smoking is rather uncommon and follows more traditional patterns. Following the Second World War, however, the appointment of women in the USSR to posts traditionally occupied by men, linked to an aspiration to equality, led to an increase in tobacco smoking in certain population groups; even so, it is still not considered acceptable for women in the USSR to smoke on public transport, in theatres and in most public places.

Statistics on the overall prevalence of smoking, while giving a broad indication of tobacco use in a population, conceal very significant differences in smoking patterns among population subgroups. In some countries, such as Spain, women have only recently begun to smoke in significant numbers, with virtually all this uptake being confined to younger women. Figure 1 illustrates that the prevalence of smoking among Spanish women below 45 years of age is of the order of 40–50%, compared with 2–5% among those aged 45 years and over. This age pattern is typical of many developed countries and points to a future epidemic of smoking-related deaths among women unless smoking cessation programmes are successful. On the other hand, the comparatively low rates of lung cancer among women in France, Portugal and Spain reflect the low prevalence of smoking among women in the past. In other countries, such as Denmark, the United Kingdom and the United States, where smoking has been common among women of all ages, lung cancer death rates are much higher.

Young women and smoking

The changing patterns of smoking among girls can be used to predict not only future patterns of tobacco-related morbidity and mortality, but also changes in smoking prevalence in the female population. The health risks associated with smoking are directly related to the age at which smoking starts and the duration of dependence (see Chapter 3). Almost a thousand million packs of cigarettes are illegally sold to youngsters in the United States each year, and it is known that the younger the age at which individuals take up smoking, the more likely it is that they will continue to smoke throughout their lives; about 90% of adult smokers take up smoking as children and adolescents.

The WHO Cross-National Survey of Health Behaviour in School-age Children, undertaken in 1986 in ten European countries (Table 8), showed a higher prevalence of smoking among

Fig. 1. Distribution of smokers by sex and age in Spain, 1987

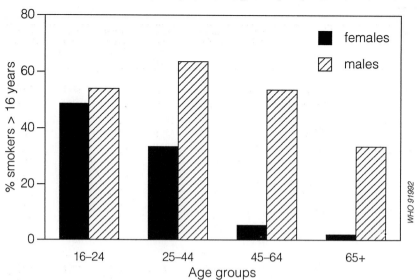

Source : National health survey, 1987.

young women (aged 15 years) than young men in five of these countries. In other countries, such as Denmark, Germany and the United States, surveys have shown higher rates of smoking among young women (aged 14–19 years) than among young men (*10*). It appears that in many countries the prevalence of smoking among girls is the same as that among boys, and what is threatening for the future is that tobacco consumption is high in both groups.

- In Finland, recent declines in smoking among teenage girls have been reversed (*11*), while in Canada in 1987, smoking prevalence was growing fastest among teenage girls (*12*).

- Among women in the United States, the average age of starting regular smoking has progressively declined with each successive birth cohort – from 35 years of age for those born before 1900, to 16 years of age among those born between 1951 and 1960 and is now virtually identical to that of young men. Every day more than 1600 American teenage girls smoke for the first time, and by 17–19 years of age, smoking prevalence among women exceeds that among men (National census).

- In the United Kingdom, the prevalence of smoking among boys was higher than among girls in 1986; in 1991 it is estimated that 27% of 15-year-old girls in England and Wales smoke compared with only 18% of boys. Since 1961 the proportion of men of all ages who smoke has fallen by more than half, to 33%; the proportion of women who smoke (30%) is now almost the same, except in Scotland where more women than men smoke. It is in the younger age groups that the changes have been greatest; 28% of women aged 16–19 years and 37% of those aged 20–24 years now smoke (*1*).

16

Table 8. Prevalence (%) of smoking among 15-year-olds in ten developed countries, 1986

Country		Smoke daily	Smoke weekly	Smoke less than weekly	Do not smoke (have tried)	Have never smoked	No. of subjects
All countries	Boys	15.0	4.4	6.5	39.9	34.2	5754
	Girls	13.8	5.6	8.0	36.2	36.3	5934
Austria	Boys	11.8	6.5	10.3	43.3	28.2	476
	Girls	13.1	7.1	11.8	39.1	28.9	381
Belgium	Boys	16.6	5.0	5.1	32.7	40.6	603
	Girls	13.5	6.2	5.6	29.4	45.3	502
Finland	Boys	29.1	6.3	6.3	39.9	18.4	539
	Girls	20.1	7.4	10.1	36.8	25.6	543
Hungary	Boys	20.4	5.9	8.2	39.9	25.4	562
	Girls	14.1	6.8	8.2	42.2	28.7	704
Israel	Boys	5.7	3.5	3.5	30.9	56.4	402
	Girls	4.1	3.4	6.3	21.3	64.9	559
Norway	Boys	16.2	4.1	9.1	43.2	27.4	627
	Girls	17.6	6.3	14.4	35.6	26.1	568
Scotland	Boys	14.7	2.6	3.6	39.8	39.2	771
	Girls	15.6	4.5	6.7	40.0	33.3	711
Sweden	Boys	8.7	5.7	7.6	47.0	31.1	541
	Girls	10.9	5.6	7.1	37.6	38.8	521
Switzerland	Boys	9.5	3.6	10.2	35.8	40.9	279
	Girls	10.5	4.4	11.3	29.3	44.4	341
Wales	Boys	13.1	2.4	4.4	41.9	38.2	954
	Girls	15.1	5.2	4.4	41.2	34.1	1104

Source: WHO Cross-National Study on Children's Health Behaviour.

It is difficult to make a more detailed comparison because of the differences in age groups surveyed and in dates of surveys. What is clear, however, is that the situation is changing rapidly and regular studies should be undertaken and publicized as such information has important implications for policies relating to tobacco control.

- In the United Kingdom, 15% of smokers aged 11 years smoked more than 26 cigarettes a week, compared with 58% of those aged 15 years; however, young men are more likely to be heavy smokers than are young women (*1*).

The use of *smokeless tobacco* (chewing tobacco and snuff) is currently rare among girls and women in developed countries. Its use by young men is relatively widespread in some developed countries, such as Sweden and the United States and the challenge

Fig. 2. Heavy smoking among young people

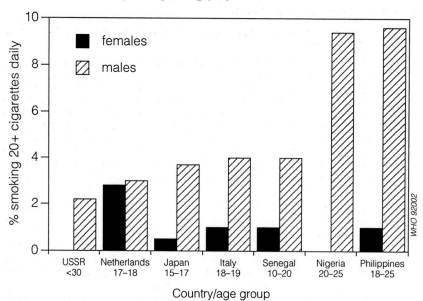

Source : Various, around 1985.

is to ensure that these forms of tobacco use are not taken up by girls.

- In Sweden the per capita smokeless tobacco consumption fell by about 75% between 1920 and 1976, but then it began to increase due to the marketing of new products (moist snuff), reflecting a marked shift in the age distribution of users. According to data obtained in 1986, moist snuff is mainly used by young people, especially young men, and has become more popular than chewing tobacco or nasal snuff. Use of these products by women remains very low (13).

- In Canada the overall usage rate for moist snuff among young people in the national population is less than 1%, but use in certain occupational, ethnic or regional groups may be many times higher than the national rate. For example, 17% of Indian girls and 20% of Indian boys aged 10–14 years use snuff (14). Snuff is less expensive than cigarettes, and appeals to children and younger teenagers, but is often replaced by cigarettes by older adolescents.

Groups at high risk

In countries where smoking has declined among women, it has become increasingly associated with economic and social disadvantages. Although smoking was first adopted by the more affluent educated women, these women were also the first to give it up. The female smoker is now more likely to have a limited education; have a lower status job or be unemployed (see Table 9); be

18

on a low income; be single, separated or divorced; or be subject to other forms of deprivation.

- In Sweden 53% of single mothers smoke compared with 26% of all adult women (15).

- Evidence from the United States shows that the narrowing gap in prevalence rates between men and women is due, in part, to higher rates of uptake of smoking among less educated young women: women without a college education are more than twice as likely to take up smoking as those who go to college (16). According to a survey conducted from 1978 to 1980, the highest rates of smoking were among cashiers (44%), machine operators (41%), nurse aides (41%), factory workers (38%), waitresses (38%), and hairdressers (37.5%). The lowest rates were among elementary school teachers (19.8%), secondary school teachers (24.8%), bank tellers (25.7%), registered nurses (27.2%), and child-care workers, excluding those in private households (28.9%).

- Studies in the United Kingdom have shown that the prevalence of smoking among women under 60 years of age is highest among those who are widowed or separated (52% in 1984 against 35% of married women), working in the home (39% against 33% of those working full-time) or unemployed (48%) (17). Table 9 shows that while smoking prevalence has decreased in all occupational groups, the figures remain higher among manual workers than other groups.

- A survey in New Zealand showed that female smokers were more likely to be in manual or unskilled occupations, have family problems or depressive symptoms and make excessive use of other dependence-producing substances. The highest proportion of smokers in the population was among the unemployed (52% for women in 1984) and those who received social security benefits (12).

- In Canada, smoking is also affected by class and occupational factors. People of lower and manual or unskilled classes are more likely to smoke than those belonging to the middle and upper classes. About 25% of female teenagers use tobacco every day, and almost 40% of women in their early twenties; prevalence rates are slightly higher than for teenage boys and young men. While 28% of employed women smoke, the rate rises to 40% for the unemployed. More smokers (women and

Table 9. Prevalence of smoking among women by socioeconomic group in the United Kingdom, 1973–86

Year	Percentage of women smokers					
	Professional	Employers and managers	Clerical and administrative workers	Skilled manual workers	Semi-skilled manual workers	Unskilled manual workers
1973	33	38	38	47	42	42
1976	28	35	36	42	41	38
1980	21	33	34	43	39	41
1984	15	29	28	37	37	36
1986	19	27	27	36	35	33

Source: reference 17.

men) are found in clerical and service occupations than in the other sectors (*18*).

- In Australia also, smoking rates are higher among the unemployed, and manual or unskilled workers than among clerical or administrative workers, for both women and men (*6*).

It has also been found that ethnicity and race may lead to social and economic disadvantages, which in turn have been associated with higher smoking rates among women.

- In New Zealand, Maori women and men smoke more than the white women and men; they are also among the poorest people in New Zealand and have one of the world's highest smoking rates for women. In Canada, a study on Indians in north-western Ontario showed that over half of the population smoked; among the women aged 15–24 years, almost 70% were smokers.
- In the Northwest Territories, the prevalence of smoking among Inuit girls was 61%; among Inuit adults the figure was 93%, and was higher in women than men (*12*). However, in the United Kingdom, white women smoke more than black women, while Asian women smoke very little (*10*).

Developing countries

On a world scale, tobacco consumption is increasing by 2.1% per annum. In developing countries tobacco consumption is increasing by about 3.4% per annum, while in developed countries it is decreasing by 0.2% per annum. Because of technological changes in the manufacture of cigarette tobacco, the changes in the number of cigarettes smoked are far greater than these percentages would indicate. In many developing countries, although sufficient information on trends and socioeconomic factors related to smoking among women may not always be available, it has been estimated that 2–10% of women smoke; in general, the prevalence of smoking among women in these countries remains low compared with that among men or with that among women in developed countries. There is an indication that in some developing countries, smoking among women is increasing and it is likely, as a result of accelerating international trade in tobacco products and the introduction of new types and flavours of cigarettes, together with the related advertising and marketing, that there will be further increases in the future.

The challenge facing developing countries is to prevent smoking from reaching the scale found in developed countries, particularly because increased tobacco consumption threatens to undo much of the progress made in health development for women. For women in developing countries, with low rates of tobacco use, it may still be possible to avoid a future epidemic and the associated

20

social and economic costs of further avoidable premature deaths and ill health caused by tobacco.

Evolution of tobacco use among women

In the majority of developing countries, smoking by women has been considered to be socially unacceptable; in some countries, a woman's smoking might even bring shame upon her father or her partner, thus reducing his social standing. However, there have always been small areas in which these restrictions did not apply and where women's smoking behaviour was similar to that of men, for example in certain areas of India, Nepal, Papua New Guinea, and northern Thailand.

In some regions where women smoke, their smoking behaviour is different from that of men. For example, in certain parts of India the practice of reverse smoking has been more prevalent among women than among men. In sub-Saharan Africa, smoking behaviour can vary between different tribes; thus in Kenya women belonging to the Masai, Samburu, Kisii and Kikuyu tribes are non-smokers but among the Luo tribe, more women than men are smokers. In the Arab world, smoking by women differs from one area to another: in many of the countries, women may smoke hubble-bubble at family gatherings or at all-women social gatherings. In some of the countries, however, they do not admit to smoking at all.

Throughout the developing world, there is often a sharp distinction between the smoking behaviour of the rural populations and that of the urban populations. Those living in the towns and cities have largely abandoned the traditional methods of using tobacco in favour of cigarettes. In some developing countries, cigarette smoking is now an activity of the younger, educated and more affluent women, usually in large cities, while older women in rural areas have retained the traditional ways of using tobacco.

The pattern and level of smoking among women in developing countries are also varied. Although the prevalence and intensity of smoking may be lower, the average tar and nicotine levels of cigarettes sold in developing countries are usually higher than in developed countries. Women's consumption of tobacco will be influenced by the fact that they generally have less access to already scarce financial resources, and are constrained by traditional and cultural factors, as well as social norms and beliefs in many countries.

- A questionnaire survey in Morocco showed a very low rate of smoking (9.8%) among devout Muslims aged 14–65 years, with a minimal rate among women (0.4%) (4).

21

The age of starting to smoke is also different from developed countries, and in some developing countries, young women are less likely than young men to be heavy smokers (i.e. smoke 20 or more cigarettes a day). While in many developed countries there is a slower rate of decline of smoking among women and in some cases, more teenage girls than teenage boys smoke, in developing countries rates for young women are usually low.

- In Costa Rica, there is evidence to suggest that women are starting to smoke at younger ages (*19*).
- In rural areas of the Islamic Republic of Iran it is not acceptable for young women to smoke but there is less stigma attached to smoking by older women, such as hubble-bubble smoking.

While smoking by women is often socially unacceptable, tobacco chewing is more widely accepted and the prevalence of chewing is surprisingly high among women in many developing countries. In Kenya, the prevalence of tobacco chewing among the women in the Masai, Samburu and Luo tribes is high at all ages and tobacco is also chewed by the older women in the Kikuyu tribe. Tobacco chewing is also fairly common among women in south-east Asia, where it may be combined with reverse smoking.

Regional patterns

Vast differences in sociocultural behaviour occur between regions and are reflected in the wide variations in patterns of tobacco consumption among women. However, all the patterns and trends point to a forthcoming serious problem.

Africa

It is currently estimated that only about 10% of women in Africa smoke, but rates are increasing, especially in urban areas. In rural areas a limiting factor is cash resources and, away from the towns, fewer women smoke and the intensity of smoking by women is usually lower; however, tobacco chewing is not uncommon. The situation in both rural and urban areas may be changing.

- In 1973, fewer than 3% of Nigerian women students smoked, but by 1982 the figure had reached 24% among female university and polytechnic students, and 52% among female trainee teachers. These students may now be in positions in which they will set an example to the community at large (*20*).

- In the early 1980s, 0.75–5.9% of women in Ghana smoked (21); in Swaziland, the prevalence rates were 3%, 4% and 7% for smokers, occasional smokers and ever smokers,[1] respectively (22). Among students in secondary and tertiary education institutions in Zambia, 4% of the women were smokers, but in the general population 7–10% of women were daily smokers (23). Among medical and paramedical students in 1983 in the Gondar College of Medical Sciences, Ethiopia, 3% of women were smokers, a rate similar to that found among the women in a Nigerian nursing school (8%) (24, 25).

As would be expected, smoking behaviours vary between the different African countries and between the different areas or tribes within those countries. In Zambia, the conventional methods of using tobacco (cigarette, cigar and pipe) are common in urban settings, but traditional methods (snuff and mishanga) remain popular in the rural areas. Such patterns probably exist in most of the African countries and it is also likely that, within many of the countries, there will be tribal differences similar to those found in Kenya (see p. 21).

In only a few of the African countries have there been any surveys of smoking in the general population; the few surveys reported tend to have been carried out on specific groups such as students. These can, however, be useful in forecasting future trends. The level of development, the degree of urbanization and the extent of penetration of life-styles which the young feel a need to emulate if they are to be considered sophisticated or successful, are all factors that are leading to an increase in the adoption of smoking in many African countries, particularly among educated and affluent women.

The information on incidence and mortality from smoking-related diseases is also limited; however, it suggests that the level of smoking by women is not insignificant and is increasing.

- In Mauritius, the number of deaths from three smoking-related cancers (cancers of the lung, larynx and oral cavity), calculated as a percentage of total cancer deaths, has increased over the period 1969–86: from 6% to 10% for women and from 19% to 29% for men. The standardized lung cancer death rates at ages 35–69 in 1960–64 were 20.6 per 100 000 for men and 2.8 per 100 000 for women. By 1985, these had increased to 37.3 per 100 000 for men and 9.0 per 100 000 for women. A male:female ratio of 7:1 in 1960 and 4:1 in 1985, suggests that women are increasingly taking up smoking. By 1987 the ratio had become 3.5:1 (26).

---

[1] Defined as people who have smoked at any time, including in the past.

Latin America

Information about the prevalence of smoking has not been systematically available for most countries in Latin America and the Caribbean.

In 1971, the Pan American Health Organization (PAHO) conducted a survey in 8 cities in Latin America to determine age-adjusted smoking prevalence rates for adult women and men. The prevalence of smoking among women ranged from 7% to 26% (compared with 30% among women in the United States), being higher among women in countries of the southern cone and the Andean subregion, than among those in Central America, Mexico and Peru. In all cities, women began to smoke at older ages and had a lower prevalence rate than men, although the difference was less marked in cities with higher levels of tobacco consumption. In most cities, the age-adjusted prevalence of cigarette smoking among women increased with higher levels of educational attainment.

Almost 150 surveys of smoking behaviour have been conducted in the past 20 years in Latin America and the Caribbean. Unfortunately, these surveys differ considerably in their sampling methods, target populations, definitions, weighting procedures and reporting formats, thus comparisons are difficult and should be interpreted with caution.

Overall, the results of the recent surveys show wide variations in the prevalence of smoking among women in Latin America, from 3% in La Paz, Bolivia, to 49% in Buenos Aires, Argentina.

The prevalence rates among women are usually lower than those among men, and are generally between 10% and 39%. Most reports of recent surveys indicate that the prevalence among women is increasing. In general, prevalence rates are lower in the less developed, predominantly rural areas and higher in countries that have undergone modernization, such as Argentina, Brazil, Chile and Uruguay, where almost as many women as men smoke.

Prevalence appears to be higher among young men than among young women and higher in the urban areas of the more developed countries of the region. Smoking among young people appears to be more common in the non-Latin Caribbean than in Central America, Mexico, and the Latin Caribbean. The prevalence of smoking among adolescents is high in some areas, and may even exceed that among adults. Almost half of the surveys reported a prevalence of greater than 30% for young men, and almost one-third reported a prevalence of greater than 30% for young women.

24

Surveys of women of childbearing age have been conducted in some countries in Latin America. The prevalence of smoking varies considerably: one-quarter of the surveys reported a prevalence of more than 30%, and more than half reported a prevalence of greater than 20%.

Although many social and demographic changes have occurred in Latin America and the Caribbean over the past two decades, four main factors may have contributed to the increase in prevalence of cigarette smoking in the region, namely:

— aging of the population;
— increasing urbanization;
— greater access to education;
— entry of women into lucrative employment.

• Thus in Costa Rica, 24% of the affluent urban women are smokers compared with only 10% of the poorer rural women (*19*). There is a trend towards smoking by younger age groups and this was also seen in Chile where, among high school students (mean age 16 years) in Santiago, 57% of boys and 59% of girls were smokers, 85% of them smoking up to 40 cigarettes per week (*3*).

South-east Asia

Cigarette consumption by women in south-east Asia appears to be very low. It is more or less static overall, measured on a per capita basis: there may have been a slight increase in smoking prevalence in one country (Thailand) and a small decrease in another (India), but overall the change is limited. However, in most south-east Asian countries, cigarettes represent only a small part of tobacco use. Thus, in assessing the health effects of tobacco, other forms of tobacco use should be taken into account, such as smoking the kretek, bidi, chutta, dhumti, khi yo, ya muan, chilum and the water pipe, and the widespread practice of tobacco chewing: gazare, khaini, naswar, zarda, and pan masala.

When every type of tobacco use is taken into account, the per capita consumption patterns look very different, showing a much higher level than is seen when cigarettes only are considered. While smoking, particularly cigarette smoking, is predominantly practised by men, chewing is very common among women. In some areas of south-east Asia, such as in some parts of rural India and in Nepal, women smoke bidis and chutta, often in reverse smoking. Similarly, pan chewing and the use of mishri (masheri) are very common in many areas of the Indian subcontinent, being used by as many as 38–59% of women, and in Andhra Pradesh, reverse smoking of chutta is considered more "feminine" than the non-reversed chutta smoked by men.

25

- In Nepal, approximately 60% of the women smoke bidis (*10*). A study in two hill villages in Nepal (1983–84) showed that 62.4% of females smoked every day. A previous study of the rural area around Kathmandu (1980) had found that 60.6% of females smoked daily (*3*).

- In Bangladesh, smoking by women is limited by poverty, customs and beliefs, although bidi smoking is common among poor rural women (*10*).

- In Indonesia, the main form of smoking is the kretek. Although smoking by women is not common, it has increased from 3.1% in 1980 to 3.9% in 1986; among primary school girls, 10% were recorded as being smokers (*27*).

- In India, the prevalence of smoking among female students was 2–5% in the early 1980s. No figures are available for the urban population, but it is estimated that no more than 5% of women are smokers. There are a number of well-defined areas in India where men, women and children all use tobacco. In Kerala, women chew tobacco; in Bihar, they smoke bidis, cheroots and hookah; in Goa, dhumti; in Maharashtra, Gujarat and Bihar, kaini, or something similar; and in Andhra, chutta in reverse smoking. In areas where women smoke there is usually an equal number of male and female smokers (*28*).

Eastern Mediterranean

The prevalence of smoking among women in the Region is affected by cultural issues, and smoking is still considered to be vulgar, improper and immoral.

- Several surveys have been conducted in Egypt, which showed that the prevalence of smoking among women and men was 0.9% and 39.8% respectively in 1978–79 and 1.5% and 32.5% in 1979–81 (*29*). In 1986, the prevalence rates were 1.0% and 39.8% and in a smaller-scale survey in 1988, the rates were 2.3% and 30.7% respectively (*30*).

- In Morocco a recent survey has shown that in secondary schools, only 8.6% of female students are smokers compared with 33% of male students. These rates are slightly increased at university level, with 10.9% of young women and 44.3% of young men smoking; the average rate (in urban areas) is 14.9% for women and 58.2% for men. Furthermore, a survey of adults working in towns (Table 10) has show that the prevalence rate is highest among women who are doctors or other professionals (*4*).

Table 10. Prevalence of smoking among adults working in towns in Morocco

Profession	Prevalence (%)		
	Men	Women	Average
Various professions	58.2	14.9	52.1
Medical doctors	53.0	25.6	50.0
Paramedical personnel	57.6	9.3	30.0

Source: reference *4*.

26

In the Gulf region, a recent survey has shown that about 8% of women and 33% of men are smokers. It was also found that smoking prevalence was high among professional and expatriate women.

Western Pacific

Throughout the Region there are wide variations in smoking behaviour, which relate to ethnic origins, geographical areas, urban/rural differences, and the degree to which western life-styles have penetrated the cultures. The prevalence of smoking among women in the Region appears to be less than 10%, except in certain rural areas of Papua New Guinea, where the prevalence is 80%. However, the overall prevalence among women is increasing because of the increasing number of schoolgirls who are taking up smoking.

- A survey of schoolchildren in Manila, Philippines in 1984 (31) found that 19% of the girls were smokers; thus smoking among women in Manila could now be at this level. Similarly, a survey of schoolchildren in Tahiti in 1979 found that the prevalence of smoking was slightly higher among girls (22%) than among boys, and this pattern could now be reflected in the adult population of the area (32).

- In many of the small Pacific island communities, the prevalence of smoking among women showed marked variations, but was seldom less than 20% (5).

- The largest country of the Region, China, could be expected to display a wide range of patterns. A survey of schoolchildren in "key" schools and in ordinary schools was reported in 1982. (Key schools are schools with the best student grades, best teachers and highest rate of students proceeding to higher education). In the ordinary schools, smoking by girls ranged from 0.4% at 12–13 years to 1.1% at 16–17 years. In the key schools, the rate was zero throughout. A household survey in Shanghai County, published in 1982, reported an overall prevalence of 2.6% among women aged 15–70 years, with the highest rate (11.6%) in the age range 60–69 years. In this survey, only 44% of men were smokers, which contrasts with the rate of 95% reported for a rural area near Guangzhou; however, there was no indication whether the female smoking prevalence was also higher in this area. Information received recently by WHO (1991) from the National Patriotic Health Campaign Committee gives the results of a 1984 survey of the population over 15 years of age. Smoking prevalence for men was given as 60% and for women the figure was 7%. The prevalence among women increased with increasing age and was higher among "workers" than among those in professional occupations (2).

- A recent survey in Hong Kong found that the prevalence of smoking among both children and adults was higher in industrialized and densely populated urban areas than more residential areas. Among grade 3 and 4 children (8–11 year olds) 10.2% of boys had tried smoking compared with 5.7% of girls (33).

27

• Anti-smoking activities have been in evidence in Singapore since the 1970s and they appear to have had some success. A survey in a low-income community with a demographic structure reflecting that of the Singapore population as a whole, carried out in 1978, showed that the prevalence of smoking was 6.3% among women and 44.3% among men. In 1984, the rates had fallen to 34.9% among men and 3.4% among women, and by 1988 were lower still at 24.6% among men and 2.4% among women. Although smoking is now declining in Singapore, the high levels of the early 1980s are still having their effect in an increasing lung cancer rate for both men and women. It is interesting to note that the smoking prevalence rates in different ethnic groups in 1978 (Chinese 45%, Malay 13% and Indian 6%) are reflected in the age-standardized lung cancer rates per 100 000: for men, Chinese 64.4, Malay 21.3, and Indian 13.1; and for women, Chinese 18.9, Malay 6.7, and Indian 7.4 (*4*).

Monitoring the epidemic

The global and regional smoking patterns presented above show that urgent action to control the smoking epidemic is needed in developing as well as developed countries.

The prevalence of tobacco smoking among women is well documented in most developed countries, as are the history and trends of smoking among women. Data on tobacco consumption and consequent ill health are comparatively rare in developing countries and more information on prevalence patterns and trends would greatly enhance the efficacy of any intervention.

Data produced by various countries are difficult to compare, and will remain so for some time as the tools for the collection of the information have not yet been standardized. In the special case of surveys on tobacco consumption by women, as already mentioned, care must be taken to ensure that prevalence data are not distorted by cultural norms or the acceptability of smoking by women in certain societies.

Confronted with the lack of information, and the diversity of the available data, and in response to a request by the World Health Assembly to monitor and report regularly on the progress and effectiveness of Member States' tobacco control programmes, WHO designed and circulated a summary country profile on the subject. This profile addresses tobacco consumption and prevalence, together with tobacco-related mortality and morbidity and other issues essential for the development and evaluation of tobacco control programmes. Section 1 of this profile outlines the "ideal" information on tobacco consumption, prevalence and intensity that should be collected at intervals of one or two years if possible. The profile, which is reproduced in Annex 1, can be used as a basis for collecting information on tobacco use by women and monitoring its effects.

Chapter 3

Tobacco or health[1]

Tobacco is a unique consumer product because of the number of deaths and diseases to which it is directly linked as a causal factor. The effects of tobacco consumption have been extensively documented for developed countries and to a lesser extent for developing countries. It is now clear that smoking-related diseases have become "equal opportunity" diseases, affecting women and men in similar ways, if they have similar exposure to tobacco and smoking behaviour. Furthermore, women have additional specific risks related to reproduction. Smoking also contributes to poverty and malnutrition.

Constituents of tobacco

The different ways in which tobacco is used have been examined in Chapter 2. The biological and health effects of tobacco consumption, including dependence, are caused by its various constituents.

Constituents of tobacco smoke

When a cigarette is smoked, a large number of chemical compounds are formed at the burning end, which are either inhaled through the cigarette as mainstream smoke, or are emitted into the air as sidestream smoke.

---

[1] Information and data presented in this chapter are based on many published studies (see references on pp. 103–106), and on unpublished evidence available to the International Agency for Research on Cancer and the World Health Organization.

Tobacco smoke is an aerosol, consisting of a particulate phase, composed of liquid droplets, dispersed in a gas/vapour phase. It contains a large variety of compounds, some 4000 of which have been identified and many have been quantified. Many of the major classes of organic chemical compounds are represented; these compounds could also be classed by their effects on the body tissues, as chemical asphyxiants, irritants, ciliastatic compounds, carcinogens, cocarcinogens or pharmacologically active compounds; some have several effects.

The aerosol particles in mainstream smoke vary in size from 0.15 μm to 1.3 μm, with a mean value of 0.4 μm. In sidestream smoke the particles are smaller, varying from 0.01 μm to 0.1 μm. Thus, the particles, the vapour phase constituents and the permanent gases can all reach the alveoli when inhaled and, indeed, it has been shown that smoke reaches every part of the trachea, bronchi and lungs and smoke constituents have been found to have been phagocytosed by alveolar macrophages.

Cancers of the trachea, bronchus and lung are caused by the deposition of carcinogens in these tissues. Some carcinogens are absorbed by the lungs and transported to other parts of the body, where they initiate cancer in other tissues.

Various diseases, grouped under the collective title of chronic obstructive pulmonary disease (COPD), arise from the smoke constituents which cause ciliastasis, produce hypersecretion and changes in the chemical structure and physical nature of mucus, irritate the bronchi and bronchioles, and cause inflammation of the membranous bronchioles.

The cardiovascular and cerebrovascular diseases are caused by the many smoke constituents that pass through the lungs and dissolve in the blood, affecting the haemoglobin, platelets, vascular tissues and heart rate.

Constituents of smokeless tobacco

At least 2500 chemical constituents of unburnt tobacco have been identified. These include, in addition to compounds derived from the tobacco itself, many substances that are added to the tobacco during cultivation, harvesting and processing. Many of the major classes of organic chemical compounds are represented and among these are many with biological activity detrimental to health, such as irritants, carcinogens and psychoactive substances, the principal representative of the latter being nicotine.

Nicotine dependence[1]

Nicotine, an alkaloid, is a constituent of all tobacco products and is fundamentally the reason why people use tobacco: nicotine-free tobacco does not satisfy the needs of those who are dependent on tobacco.

Alkaloids are a group of chemical compounds of plant origin, many of which have long been used by people for their medicinal properties, their psychoactive effects and as poisons. Most alkaloids are poisonous at high concentrations and nicotine is no exception; at high exposure levels it is a potent and lethal poison.

Alkaloids are by definition alkali-like and nicotine can exist as the free base or as a salt. When tobacco is combined with lime for chewing, as in south-east Asia, the nicotine is released from the tobacco as the free base, and absorbed in the mouth. Smoke from pipes and cigars also contains nicotine as the free base which is absorbed in the mouth and nose. The smoke from other nicotine-delivery devices, particularly cigarettes, is acidic; in this case, the nicotine is absorbed in the lungs.

The absorption of nicotine by the blood is very rapid; nicotine is quickly distributed to the brain and its effects on the central nervous system are manifested almost instantaneously.

Studies in both humans and animals have shown that nicotine is a potent psychoactive drug. High doses can lead to intoxication and death; at doses typically obtained from tobacco products, nicotine is responsible for much of the pleasure and satisfaction obtained by tobacco users. Through activation of nicotine receptors in the central nervous system, nicotine can produce dependence. It also appears that nicotine can alleviate various dysphoric states associated with boredom, stress, and the nicotine withdrawal syndrome.

Nicotine administration can lead to tolerance and physiological dependence. Tolerance is indicated by the diminished response to repeated doses of nicotine. Nicotine-induced physiological dependence and withdrawal are specific to the administration or removal of nicotine itself. The withdrawal syndrome includes a craving for nicotine, impaired ability to concentrate, disrupted cognitive performance, mood changes, and impaired brain function. The severity of the symptoms may be such that heavy smokers are unable to abstain permanently from tobacco without treatment; however, the symptoms usually disappear within a few weeks.

---

[1] This section is based on information received from Dr J. Henningfield, Chief, Clinical Pharmacology Branch, National Institute on Drug Abuse, Addiction Research Center, Baltimore, MD, USA.

Nicotine dependence, like other forms of drug dependence, is a progressive, chronic, relapsing disorder. The severity of the disorder varies from low levels to levels at which the behaviour is highly resistant to change.

Mortality and morbidity

In 1980 the report of the US Surgeon-General on *The health consequences of smoking for women* (*34*) exposed clearly the fallacy of the belief that women were immune to tobacco-related diseases. This impression was gained from studies conducted between 1950 and 1980, which compared the death rates from tobacco-related diseases among men with those among women. More recent research has shown that whenever the cigarette smoking characteristics — in particular duration and intensity — of women emulate those of men, their relative risks of smoking-related illness are likely to be similar.

Currently, tobacco use is estimated to account for 3 million deaths per year. More than half of these occur in developed countries, and more than 300 000 of them are among women in these countries. The cumulative exposure of women to tobacco (primarily from smoking) has been much higher in these countries than in the developing countries and as a consequence the death rates from smoking-related diseases among women in developing countries are likely still to be relatively low. However, the mortality rates from other forms of tobacco use among women (primarily chewing) is substantially higher in developing countries, with annual estimates of at least 100 000 deaths in India alone. Current trends suggest that among women who smoke, at least 25% will die from smoking-related diseases.

In Chapter 2, it was pointed out that the uptake and increase in tobacco consumption by women is mainly in the form of smoking, particularly cigarette smoking; consequently this chapter will concentrate on this issue. However, in some developing countries such as India, cigarette smoking represents only a small fraction of the total tobacco consumption, in particular among women in rural areas. In these countries, smokeless tobacco is also imposing its burden of tobacco-related diseases and deaths. The risks of oral cancer, as well as of numerous odontological disorders and diseases of the mouth and gums, are greatly increased by the use of smokeless tobacco. Smokeless tobacco use has also been shown to be related to hypertension and an increased heart rate. In addition, tobacco chewing poses specific risks for women, e.g. for potential adverse effects on the fetus during pregnancy.

34

Fig. 3. Estimated distribution of deaths from various smoking-related diseases among women in developed countries, 1985

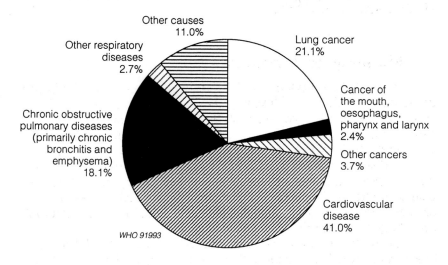

Total 300 000 deaths

In countries where smoking is a long-established custom, about 90% of lung cancer cases, 30% of all cancers, and over 80% of cases of chronic bronchitis and emphysema are attributable to tobacco use, as are some 20–25% of deaths from coronary heart disease and stroke. In countries where smokeless tobacco use has been predominant, such as in the Indian subcontinent, it is a major cause of oral cancer.

An overview of the principal causes of smoking-related deaths among women in the developed countries for which reliable mortality statistics are available is given in Fig. 3. Of the 300 000 deaths attributable to smoking among women in these countries in 1985, 21.1% were coded to lung cancer, 41% to cardiovascular diseases, primarily coronary heart disease and stroke, and 18.1% to chronic obstructive pulmonary disease. The proportionate distribution was similar for men.

In 1980 the US Surgeon-General made the following comments about women smokers in the United States, which can also be expected to apply in other countries: "Women demonstrate the same dose-response relationships with cigarette smoking as men. An increase in mortality occurs with an increase in the number of cigarettes smoked per day, an earlier age of beginning cigarette smoking, a longer duration of smoking, inhalation of cigarette smoke, and a higher tar and nicotine content of the cigarette. Women who have smoking characteristics similar to men may experience mortality rates similar to men'' (*34*).

- A recent study which examined the life expectancies of cigarette smokers and non-smokers in the United States found that women and men who are heavy smokers at 25 years of age can expect at least a 25% shorter life than non-smokers (*35*).

A summary of the relative risks[1] for smokers in the United States for various causes of death is given in Table 11. In addition to the gender differences, Table 11 demonstrates how the risks for women multiplied over the two decades between the two studies, commensurate with their longer exposure to smoking. This is particularly evident for lung cancer, where the relative risk increased almost fivefold to a level similar to that found for men in the 1960s. A similar pattern is found in most developed countries and is likely to emerge in a growing number of developing countries as exposure to tobacco increases.

Table 11. Summary of estimated relative risks for various causes of death among current cigarette smokers aged 35 years and older, Cancer Prevention Study, 1959–65 (CPS-I) and 1982–86 (CPS-II)

Underlying cause of death	Men		Women	
	CPS-I	CPS-II	CPS-I	CPS-II
Coronary heart disease, age 35	1.83	1.94	1.40	1.78
Coronary heart disease, age 35–64	2.25	2.81	1.81	3.00
Cerebrovascular lesions, age 35	1.37	2.24	1.19	1.84
Cerebrovascular lesions, age 35–64	1.79	3.67	1.92	4.80
Chronic obstructive pulmonary disease	8.81	9.65	5.89	10.47
Cancer of the lips, oral cavity, and pharynx	6.33	27.48	1.96	5.59
Oesophageal cancer	3.62	7.60	1.94	10.25
Pancreatic cancer	2.34	2.14	1.39	2.33
Laryngeal cancer	10.00	10.48	3.81	17.78
Lung cancer	11.35	22.36	2.69	11.94

Source: reference *36*.

[1] Relative risk describes the risk of dying or developing a disease for a person exposed to a particular risk factor (in this case cigarette smoking) compared with someone not exposed.

Estimates of relative risks are not available for women in developing countries, but current rates of tobacco-related diseases are likely to be generally lower than in developed countries as relatively few women smoked until recently. Since there is a definite time-lag between the onset of smoking and the development of smoking-related diseases, such as lung cancer and heart disease, the number of tobacco-related deaths among women in both developed and developing countries is likely to increase well into the next century.

Tobacco consumption is also an important cause of morbidity, affecting the quality of life of women, either as sufferer or carer for other family members affected by tobacco-related diseases. Ill health arises from numerous tobacco-related conditions, including respiratory distress, gastric ulcers and pregnancy complications. The adverse effects of smoking on pregnancy range from low birth weight to increased incidence of spontaneous abortions, premature births, stillbirths and neonatal deaths. Low birth weight is one of the strongest predictors of infant mortality.

Tobacco smoke is not only dangerous to the smoker but to nearby non-smokers as well. Besides the acute effects of eye and throat irritation due to exposure to the smoke, passive smoking is detrimental to the respiratory tissues and increases the risk of lung cancer and cardiovascular disease in non-smokers. Children are particularly vulnerable to the damaging effects of enforced passive smoking.

Thus, in the case of women it is not enough to consider only the direct effects of tobacco consumption because, in most societies, they are also the primary carers of children and their smoking puts these children directly at risk, as well as providing role models of smoking to children. Parental smoking may also have economic consequences and repercussions on the child's well-being (e.g. fewer resources may be available to purchase food).

Cardiovascular diseases

Among the causes of death related to tobacco use, cardiovascular diseases represent the most important absolute risk. Both nicotine and carbon monoxide are contributory or supportive factors in the development of coronary artery and peripheral vascular disease. In many developed countries, there have been dramatic falls in mortality from these diseases due largely to a reduction in risk factors, including smoking cessation. Further reductions in mortality are possible with further decline in smoking.

37

Coronary heart disease

Coronary heart disease (CHD), including acute myocardial infarction (heart attack) and chronic ischaemic heart disease, is more common in women who smoke than in those who are non-smokers. Cigarette smoking increases the risk of CHD by approximately twofold, and in younger women it may increase the risk several-fold. Cigarette smoking also acts synergistically with other CHD risk factors, producing a risk greater than the sum of all the individual risks.

Overall, the death rate from CHD among smokers is 80–90% greater than among non-smokers, equivalent to a 2–4-fold greater risk of sudden death. The risk of myocardial infarction is multifactorial. The presence of one or more of the major CHD risk factors, such as cigarette smoking, hyper-cholesterolaemia, and hypertension puts individuals at high or very high risk. The risk of CHD is also increased among diabetic smokers and among smokers with genetic familial hyperlipidaemias.

Studies in North America, northern Europe and Japan have shown that cigarette smokers are at greater risk than non-smokers for fatal and non-fatal myocardial infarction and for sudden death. Women who smoke and use oral contraceptives are on average about 5–10 times more likely to develop heart disease than those who use the pill and do not smoke. This risk increases with age, and is particularly high among women over 40 years. The estimated risk of myocardial infarction among current smokers also increases with the number of cigarettes smoked daily and does not depend on either the nicotine or carbon monoxide yield of the cigarette. In other words, the risk of CHD is *not* reduced by smoking cigarettes with a lower tar and nicotine yield. This is particularly important for women who may smoke these cigarettes, thinking them to be safer.

However, there is clear evidence that giving up smoking markedly reduces the risk of dying from heart disease or stroke. This decline in risk is evident soon after giving up smoking and continues with time. There is thus considerable scope for further marked declines in mortality and morbidity from CHD among women as smoking cessation programmes become more effective.

Cerebrovascular disease

In populations where women have smoked for several decades, it is estimated that smoking accounts for approximately 55% of deaths from cerebrovascular disease in women under

38

65 years. The two major types of cerebrovascular disease (collectively known as "stroke") are: (a) cerebral infarction, and (b) cerebral haemorrhage. Cigarette smoking makes a significant, independent contribution to the risk of stroke, which increases with the number of cigarettes smoked. Use of both the pill and cigarettes synergistically increases the risk of cerebral haemorrhage in women.

Until recently, the relationship between cigarette smoking and the risk of stroke had been unclear. Recent studies have now confirmed that smoking is an important independent risk factor for stroke in both women and men and that the risk decreases on cessation of smoking. The risk of stroke among women smokers is highest among middle-aged women and stroke is therefore responsible for a significant number of premature deaths among women smokers.

Atherosclerosis

While the incidence of peripheral vascular disease is increased among all smokers, the condition is more common in men than in women. There is a significant association between cigarette smoking and atherosclerosis, cigarette smoking being directly related to the extent of atherosclerotic disease involving large and small arteries in the lower extremities. Diabetes mellitus and cigarette smoking are key risk factors for arterial disease of the lower extremities and the cause of many amputations.

Aortic aneurysm

Cigarette smoking has been associated with an increased risk of aortic aneurysm. The mortality rate from abdominal aortic aneurysm among cigarette smokers (male and female) is 2–8 times the rate among non-smokers.

Hypertension

Cigarette smoking has also been associated with low serum levels of high-density lipoprotein and hypertension. Smoking by patients with hypertension is an important disease risk factor; the risk of coronary heart disease and stroke is 50–60% higher in smokers with high blood pressure than in non-smokers with high blood pressure.

Cancer

Each year, it is estimated that about 6.5 million new cases of cancer occur throughout the world, with about half of them occurring in men and half in women. For women, the most common cancers are breast cancer, cervical cancer, colorectal cancer, stomach cancer and lung cancer, in that order. Among men, lung cancer is most common (reflecting their longer and more extensive exposure to tobacco than women), followed by stomach cancer, colorectal cancer, cancer of the mouth and pharynx and prostate cancer.

In developed countries, smoking is estimated to cause about 85 000 cancer deaths a year among women or approximately 8% of all deaths from cancer among women. Among men, over 500 000 cancer deaths a year or just over 40% of all cancer deaths are attributable to smoking. The proportions are undoubtedly lower in developing countries but are increasing.

- In India it is estimated that about one-fifth of all cancers in women are attributable to tobacco use (37).
- In south-east Asia, where smokeless forms of tobacco are widely used, cancers of the mouth and pharynx are twice as common as lung cancer in men and are the third most common form of cancer in women.

Lung cancer

Cigarette smoking is considered to be the major cause of lung cancer in populations where smoking has been common for many years. In developed countries, smoking is associated with about two-thirds of lung cancer cases among women; however, in the United Kingdom and United States, where women have been smoking for several decades, it is associated with about 80% of cases. Since the 1960s, there has been a steady and dramatic increase in the number of deaths from lung cancer among women; overall, death rates from lung cancer among women in developed countries increased by almost 200% between 1957 and 1987 (see Fig. 4). Lung cancer death rates in Japan, Norway, Poland, Sweden and the United Kingdom doubled, and in Australia, Denmark and New Zealand increased by 200%. In Canada and the United States, the rates increased by over 300%.

In addition to the number of deaths, the suffering experienced by cancer patients should also be recognized. Unfortunately, for most tobacco-related cancers, particularly lung cancer, the case-fatality rate (death rate among those who have the disease) is very high and survival is usually short, of only a few months' duration.

40

Fig. 4. Trends in lung cancer mortality by sex in developed countries, 1957–87

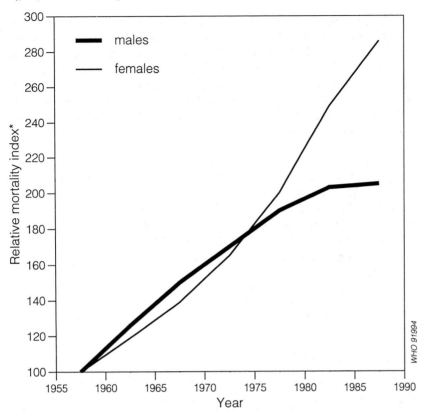

* Death rate for each period expressed as a percentage of the mortality level for 1955–59.

The risk of lung cancer among women smokers increases with the number of cigarettes smoked per day, duration of smoking behaviour, degree of inhalation, age of starting to smoke, and amount of tar (high, medium or low). In the determination of the risk of lung cancer associated with the quantity of tobacco smoked, two components can be identified: the number of cigarettes smoked per day and the duration of smoking behaviour. While an increase in either factor leads to a higher risk, the effect of the duration of smoking is greater than that of the daily consumption of tobacco.

Cigarette smoking is associated with the majority of cases of lung cancer in women and men. In addition, some cases are linked with passive smoking, while others are linked with exposure to other carcinogens, such as radon. There have been reports of an increased risk of lung cancer among coal miners and studies have

41

been conducted to examine the risk for subjects exposed to radon in their homes. Most of the increase in risk occurred among smokers. Living in houses with a high level of exposure to radon will be especially harmful to women smokers, who usually spend more time at home.

Evidence for cigarette smoking being the major cause of lung cancer mortality is provided in Fig. 5, which illustrates the sharp increase in mortality among women smokers in the United States over the period 1960–86, compared with the constant low rate among women who are non-smokers.

Fig. 5. Age-standardized death rates from lung cancer among women in the United States, 1960–86

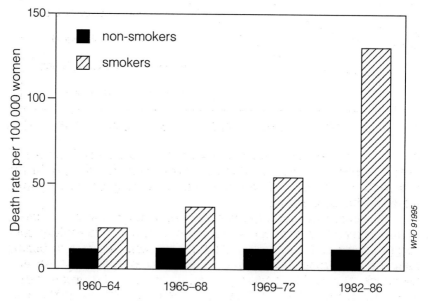

In Japan, Scotland and the United States, lung cancer now accounts for more deaths among women than breast cancer (Fig. 6). In other parts of the United Kingdom, as well as in Australia and Denmark, lung cancer mortality rates among women are reaching breast cancer mortality rates. In England and Wales, lung cancer mortality rates among women have increased by 250% since the 1970s, and have almost overtaken breast cancer in women aged 65–75 years who started smoking during the Second World War.

The trends in mortality from lung cancer among women in developed countries are shown in Table 12. Only in a few coun-

Fig. 6. Trends in age-standardized death rates from lung and breast cancer among women aged 35–74 years, Scotland and the United States, 1955–89

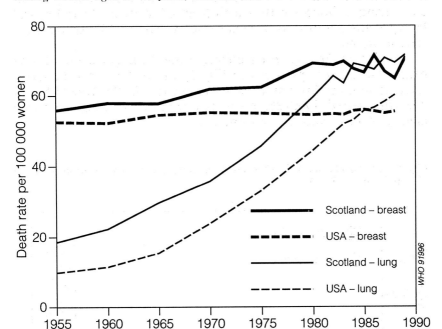

tries (France, Portugal and Spain) are lung cancer death rates still low; however, the rates in these countries will rise sharply in the near future as a result of the very significant proportions of young women who now smoke.

As more and more women die from lung cancer, the levels of mortality from the disease in some countries are rapidly converging towards those in men. As Fig. 7 shows, the male to female ratio of lung cancer death rates in countries such as Australia, Denmark, England and Wales, and the United States declined dramatically from 7–10:1 in the early 1960s to 3:1 in 1985. This trend is expected to continue as the smoking epidemic among men in these countries stabilizes or begins to decline but rates for women continue to rise.

Other cancers

Figures based on studies in the United States of America show that smoking is associated with a very significant proportion of other cancers in women, including cancer of the oral cavity (61%), oesophagus (75%), pancreas (34%), larynx (87%), bladder (37%), and kidney (12%).

Table 12. Patterns and trends of lung cancer mortality among women in developed countries, 1950–90

Country	Age-standardized[a] mortality rate from lung cancer per 100 000 population					
	1950–54	1960–64	1970–74	1975–79	1980–84	1985–90[b]
Group 1 — Mortality high and rising						
Australia	4.5	5.6	9.7	12.2	15.1	18.6
Canada	4.8	6.0	11.0	15.6	21.5	29.6
Denmark	6.1	8.7	13.7	18.2	25.0	34.4
England & Wales	8.8	12.5	19.2	22.8	26.3	30.1
Hungary	8.1[c]	10.1	12.0	13.1	15.7	20.8
Ireland	6.0	9.2	16.7	20.4	24.7	28.3
New Zealand	4.2	7.1	13.9	16.7	19.9	24.9
United States	5.7	7.4	15.1	20.4	26.9	33.9
Group 2 — Mortality intermediate and rising steadily						
Austria	8.8[c]	8.4	9.5	10.2	11.8	12.8
Belgium	5.2[c]	6.1	7.4	8.5	9.4	11.1
Czechoslovakia	7.9[c]	8.1	8.1	9.1	10.2	12.3
Germany	5.6	7.0	7.1	7.9	9.2	11.8
Italy	3.9	5.8	7.1	8.2	9.1	10.8
Japan	1.9	5.8	8.0	9.5	11.2	12.6
Netherlands	4.7	5.1	5.9	7.3	10.1	14.9
Norway	3.7	3.9	5.6	6.9	9.5	14.6
Sweden	5.4	5.6	7.9	9.3	11.3	14.2
Switzerland	4.6	4.5	5.7	6.6	8.4	10.2
Group 3 — Mortality low and rising slowly						
Finland	6.1	5.4	6.1	7.5	8.6	9.4
France	4.5	5.2	5.1	5.3	5.9	7.5
Portugal	3.1[c]	3.4	4.6	4.6	5.4	6.0
Group 4 — Mortality still on plateau						
Spain	3.4	5.2	5.9	5.8	5.6	5.5

[a] The "European" population age structure was used as the standard.
[b] Latest available year.
[c] Data refer to 1955–59.

Source: Lopez AD. Changes in tobacco consumption and lung cancer risk; evidence from national statistics. In: Hakama MM et al., ed. *Evaluating effectiveness of primary prevention of cancer.* Lyon, International Agency for Research on Cancer, 1990, pp. 53–76 (IARC Scientific Publications, No. 103).

Laryngeal cancer has recently become more common in women. Smokers are at higher risk of the disease, thus with the increased prevalence of smoking among women, an increase in the incidence of laryngeal cancer could be expected. Such a tendency may be present in a few countries, but is difficult to assess accurately because of the still low rate of the disease in women. However, the male to female ratio of laryngeal cancer death rates, which in most parts of the world is of the order of 10–20:1, is

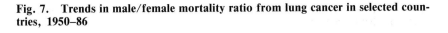

Fig. 7. Trends in male/female mortality ratio from lung cancer in selected countries, 1950–86

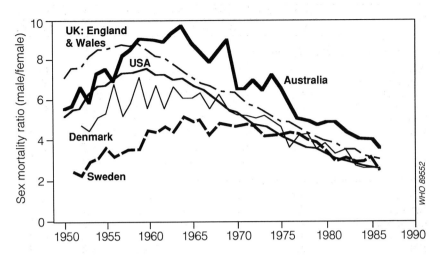

much lower (5–6:1) in countries such as Canada and the United Kingdom, where women smoked heavily in the past.

Oral cancers include cancers of the lips, tongue, gums, buccal mucosa, hard and soft palate, salivary glands, floor of the mouth and oropharynx. Oral cancer is a major problem in certain developing countries, particularly in south-east Asia, where a variety of traditional tobacco uses (e.g. chewing or smoking with the burning end of the chutta inside the mouth) are associated with 85–90% of cases among women. Cigarette, pipe and cigar smoking have all been linked to an increased risk of oral cancer. Heavy use of alcohol has been identified as an independent risk factor. The use of both tobacco and alcohol combined with poor oral hygiene or inadequate dentition also increases the risk of developing oral cancer.

Use of smokeless tobacco products (snuff and various forms of chewing tobacco) has been associated with cancers of the gingiva, mouth, lips, tongue, pharynx, larynx and oesophagus. Inhalation of snuff has also been linked to the occurrence of nasal cancer.

The highest reported incidence rate in the world for cancer of the mouth is among women in Bangalore, India, where women have considerably higher rates than men; this pattern is also found in Madras. In contrast, the incidence of lung cancer among women in these cities is extremely low. Again, this shows that when assessing the global effects of tobacco consumption, it is not sufficient to consider only cigarette consumption and lung cancer.

45

The risk of oesophageal cancer increases with the use of tobacco and alcohol. Mortality rates from the disease among pipe and cigar smokers are similar to rates among cigarette smokers.

Cigarette smoking is a risk factor for both *urinary bladder* and *kidney cancer*. Smoking compounds the risks of certain tropical diseases: the risk of bladder cancer, for example, is greater among people suffering from schistosomiasis, and β-naphthylamine contained in tobacco tar is a bladder carcinogen (*38*). Smoking also enhances the risk of bladder cancer associated with certain occupational exposures.

Cigarette smoking is closely linked to the occurrence of *pancreatic cancer*, with the risk increasing with an increase in cigarette consumption.

- Studies have shown that the mortality ratio for pancreatic cancer was 1.94 for Japanese women smokers in comparison with non-smokers, and 2–3 for women smokers in Sweden and the United States (*34, 39*).
- Studies in Japan and Sweden have shown that women who smoke are 1.6–2.7 times more likely to develop bladder cancer than those who do not smoke (*34*).

Significantly, for women, cigarette smoking has been associated with a twofold increase in the risk of *cervical cancer*. This may in part be due to confounding with other risk factors since this form of cancer is also strongly linked with certain types of sexual behaviour which might be more prevalent among smokers than non-smokers. Young women who start smoking at an early age, for example, may also become sexually active at an earlier age than those who do not smoke.

A number of studies have shown a slightly lower risk of *endometrial cancer* among women smokers. This may be due to the anti-estrogenic effect of tobacco. However, the prevalence of this type of cancer is very low and the reduction in risk is negligible compared with the greatly increased risk of other cancers associated with smoking.

Bronchopulmonary diseases

There are several bronchopulmonary disease conditions that are classified under the heading chronic obstructive pulmonary disease (COPD). Undoubtedly, smoking is the most important risk factor for COPD in developed countries, although atmospheric pollution in cities and indoor pollution from fires in houses without chimneys are major contributory factors for women in developing countries. Industrial dust and fumes in the workplace have also been implicated, but to a much lesser extent. COPD may be defined as a condition characterized by the development of airways obstruction and the presence of chronic bronchitis, bronchiolitis, emphysema or asthma. Emphysema, a major component of COPD, is an abnormal permanent enlargement of the air spaces distal to the terminal bronchioles, either from dilatation or from obstruction of their walls. Most people who die from COPD have emphysema.

> • In the United States, COPD morbidity has significantly increased in women, while it has remained almost constant in men. The trends in the prevalence of COPD — stable or downwards for men since 1980, and upwards for women — are consistent with changes in cigarette smoking among these groups (37).

Several studies have shown that respiratory conditions, such as cough, sputum, wheezing and dyspnoea (shortness of breath) are more common among smokers than among non-smokers. There is also a higher frequency of pulmonary functional abnormalities among smokers.

The prevalence of chronic bronchitis among smokers increases with the number of cigarettes smoked per day. A close relationship has been demonstrated between cigarette smoking and chronic cough or sputum production in women; these symptoms also increase with the number of packs smoked over the years.

In developed countries, COPD mortality is highest in the eastern European countries, England and Wales, Ireland, and Scotland, and is lowest in southern Europe, Israel and Japan. However, differences are difficult to quantify because of differences between countries in diagnostic and coding practices. In the past, the trend in COPD mortality has been upwards. In recent years there have been substantial declines in death rates in most countries for the major causes of death, but not for COPD or lung cancer.

> • In the United States, COPD is one of the few leading causes of death that has shown a steady increase since 1950. The trend for COPD mortality has been similar to that for lung cancer. More than 95% of COPD deaths occur in people over the age of 55. Men have appreciably higher death rates than women; however, the rate of increase has been much more rapid among women than men since 1979. Whereas men showed a 16% increase in mortality, women have experienced a 73% increase (40). It has been estimated that the smoking-attributable proportions of mortality from COPD in the USA are 84% for men and 79% for women (41).

In European countries, COPD mortality in women over 55 years is increasing. In England and Wales, the increase is about 8–9% per year; trends are also upwards for women in France, the Netherlands, and Scotland.

47

• In a Swedish study, the death rate from bronchitis, emphysema and asthma among female smokers was 2.2 times that among non-smokers; this ratio is similar to that reported for the United States (*39*).

In developing countries few reliable data are available and it is difficult to give a precise picture of the situation. In some countries, such as China and Nepal, the combination of smoking and passive smoking with exposure to domestic smoke from cooking and heating in poorly ventilated houses has been associated with an increased incidence of chronic bronchitis and cor pulmonale.

Reproductive health

Smoking is associated with increased risks of infertility. Women who smoke are more susceptible to infections of the reproductive tract and may be less fertile. For example, women who smoke more than 20 cigarettes a day are three times more likely than non-smokers to take more than a year to conceive, with three times the risk of primary tubal infertility, and a greater risk of ectopic pregnancy.

Furthermore, women who smoke and use oral contraceptives are at greater risk of cardiovascular disease than those who use the pill and do not smoke (see p. 37).

Smoking during pregnancy has been associated with premature delivery, spontaneous abortion and fetal and perinatal death. Some of the conditions present a risk for the health of the mother herself, and may occur particularly in countries where pregnant women do not generally have easy access to adequate care in the event of problems such as ectopic pregnancy, and where there is a greater incidence of anaemia among women.

In the Indian subcontinent, associations have been reported between use of smokeless tobacco during pregnancy and adverse reproductive outcome. In one study, the stillbirth rate among women who chewed tobacco during pregnancy was much higher than that among women who did not. Furthermore, the offspring of the mothers who chewed tobacco had a lower birth weight; this was associated with a decrease in the mean gestation period (*42*).

Similarly, smoking during pregnancy has been shown to increase the risk of delivering a low-birth-weight baby, independently of factors such as race, parity, maternal size, socioeconomic status, sex of child, or gestational age. There is a dose-response relationship, i.e. the more the woman smokes during pregnancy, the greater the reduction in birth weight. If the mother is able to give up smoking by the fourth month of gestation, her risk of delivering a low-birth-weight baby is similar to that of a non-smoker.

48

According to research conducted in developed countries, women who smoke have 1.2–1.8 times as many spontaneous abortions as women who are non-smokers.

- In a study at three hospitals in New York, USA, the risk of having a spontaneous abortion for regular smokers increased by 46% for the first 10 cigarettes smoked a day, and by 61% for the first 20 cigarettes (36).

Smoking is an important risk factor for perinatal death. It has been estimated in some developed countries that if all women gave up smoking, the number of fetal and infant deaths would drop by approximately 10%. The sudden infant death syndrome, a major cause of infant mortality in developed countries, has also been linked to maternal smoking during pregnancy. Mortality from this condition has been rising in several countries and in some countries, such as France, Germany and the United Kingdom, now accounts for 20–25% of all infant deaths.

- A recent survey of more than 360 000 births in Missouri, USA, and a survey of 281 000 births in Sweden, have shown that smoking plays a significant role in late fetal and early neonatal death, especially when combined with other biological risk factors, such as high maternal age and multiple births. The Swedish study suggested that smoking was responsible for 11% of late fetal deaths and 5% of early neonatal deaths (36).

In those developing countries where the health of the mother and her baby is already jeopardized because of poverty and malnutrition, these disadvantages combined with the effects of smoking will have an even greater impact on the incidence of perinatal mortality.

- In Chile it is estimated that 10% of non-accidental perinatal deaths are attributable to smoking (36).

Menstrual disorders including dysmenorrhoea, premenstrual tension, irregular menses and secondary amenorrhoea have been associated with smoking, and women who smoke typically go through the menopause two or three years earlier than non-smokers. Cigarette smoking seems to increase the risk of estrogen-deficiency diseases, such as postmenopausal osteoporosis and subsequent fractures. After the menopause, the risk of cardiovascular disease among women becomes equal to that among men.

Other effects on well-being

Nicotine reduces the circulation of blood and the uptake of oxygen, affecting not only the skin, but also the hair and the eyes. Contrary to the images of youthful and healthy women often promoted in cigarette advertising, smoking produces bad breath, gum disease, dental problems, a hoarse voice, cough, a decreased sense of smell, stained teeth and fingernails, and premature wrinkles.

Similarly, use of smokeless tobacco can stain the teeth and cause bad breath, tooth erosion, dental caries, tooth loss, a decreased sense of taste, alveolar bone destruction and gingival recession, as well as other effects on gingival and periodontal health. The healing of oral lesions has also been noted to be slower among users.

Smoking and occupational health

In addition to the direct effects caused by tobacco consumption, smoking may interact with hazardous materials in the workplace.

— Tobacco products may become contaminated with toxic agents in the workplace; they can facilitate the entry of the agent by inhalation, ingestion and skin absorption.

— Chemicals may be transformed into more harmful agents with smoking.

— Certain toxic agents in tobacco smoke may also be present at the workplace, leading therefore, to increased exposure to the agent.

— Smoking may act synergistically with toxic agents.

— Smoking can cause accidents at the workplace, for example, fires and even explosions.

Women with the same occupational exposure to environmental hazards and smoking behaviour as men are likely to develop similar health problems. Furthermore, smoking and occupational exposure may have a cumulative effect on the health of the fetus or the mother during pregnancy.

Air pollution or occupational exposures were often believed to be the main reasons for increased lung cancer mortality. While these factors have been shown to be linked to mortality from lung cancer and the occurrence of other respiratory diseases, active smoking has been shown to have a much greater effect. Indeed, in situations where there is both outdoor and indoor air pollution, active smoking multiplies the risks. In addition, active smoking is something that can be avoided; cleaning ambient air is more difficult and is a slower process.

50

Studies have shown that exposure of women to smoking and asbestos multiplies the risk of lung cancer. Women who smoke and are exposed to cotton dust have a higher risk of developing byssinosis, chronic bronchitis and chronic obstructive pulmonary disease and show abnormal effects in pulmonary function tests more often than those who do not smoke.

- A study of workers in mills producing cotton and man-made fibres in England showed that the prevalence of byssinosis among women and men who smoked was 1.4 times that among non-smokers; the risk was strongly associated with the duration of exposure to cotton dust (*34*).

Passive smoking

Passive smoking, also known as involuntary smoking or inhalation of environmental tobacco smoke, is of increasing concern because of growing awareness of its detrimental effects on health. Important considerations in examining the risks of passive smoking are the composition of environmental tobacco smoke and its toxicity and carcinogenicity.

Environmental tobacco smoke has two constituents: mainstream cigarette smoke exhaled by the smoker and sidestream smoke, the smoke emitted from the burning end of the cigarette. Comparison of the chemical composition of the smoke inhaled by active smokers with that inhaled by involuntary smokers suggests that the toxic and carcinogenic effects are qualitatively similar; however, although there is a greater dilution of sidestream smoke, greater amounts of many of the organic constituents of smoke, including some carcinogens, are found in sidestream smoke.

Exposure to environmental tobacco smoke increases the risks of disease for non-smokers. This concerns women in two respects. Firstly, women smokers are fewer in number than men smokers, both in the home and at work, and therefore larger numbers of women than men are more likely to be exposed to passive smoking. Secondly, as women are usually the primary carers of the family, children are more likely to be exposed to passive smoking if their mother smokes than if their father smokes.

According to the 1986 report of the US Surgeon-General (*39*) there is compelling evidence that :

— involuntary smoking is a cause of disease, including lung cancer, in otherwise healthy non-smokers;

— children whose parents smoke have an increased frequency of respiratory infections, increased respiratory symptoms, and slightly lower rates of increase in lung function as the lung matures than children whose parents are non-smokers;

— the simple separation of smokers and non-smokers within the same air space may reduce, but does not eliminate, the exposure of non-smokers to environmental tobacco smoke.

Health consequences for women

Women's health may be impaired by other people's tobacco smoke at home, at work or in public places. Several studies have shown that women who are non-smokers and whose partner smokes have a 20–50% greater risk of developing lung cancer than those whose partner does not smoke.

- The National Research Council report for 1986 stated that at least 2500 of the 12 000 deaths from lung cancer among non-smokers in the United States could be attributed to passive smoking. The total number of deaths from lung cancer in the United States in 1986 was about 136 000.

The effects of exposure to a partner's smoking may be manifested only after many years of exposure for cancers, but there are several more rapid detrimental effects on the heart and cardiovascular system.

- A study conducted among rural women in the USA showed that the relative risk of death from cardiovascular disease was 1.59, and 1.39 for all causes of mortality, for women whose partners smoked cigarettes compared with women whose partners were non-smokers, after adjustment for age, cholesterol, blood pressure, and body mass (43).

Women who work in the service sector often have little control over policy on smoking on the premises. Such is the case for canteen staff and most secretaries. However, it should be noted that a number of recent litigation cases in Australia, Sweden and the United Kingdom have recognized that passive smoking is an occupational hazard.

Furthermore, the effect of passive smoking on pregnant women deserves more attention. If a woman who does not smoke is exposed to tobacco smoke during pregnancy, there could be detrimental effects.

- A study in Osaka, Japan, of 3478 pregnant women showed that the prevalence rate of low birth weight increased with the intensity of exposure to tobacco smoke during pregnancy; among non-smokers, the prevalence was 3.8% for women whose partners were non-smokers, but 5.6% for women whose partners were smokers (44).

Health consequences for children

Many women are becoming more aware of the danger of smoking during pregnancy, but are unaware of the risks of smoking after delivery; few regular smokers realize that their children are passively smoking.

- In a study in Japan, schoolchildren were found to have quantities of smoke-related chemicals in the urine related to the number of cigarettes that their parents smoked at home. A study carried out in the United Kingdom had the same findings, even among children aged between 11 and 16, where the amount of cotinine in their saliva was related to the number of smokers in the family (A. Charlton, personal communication, 1991).

Children who are constantly exposed to tobacco smoke have a tendency to suffer from a series of health problems in the first few years of life, especially respiratory illnesses and infections. A higher incidence of pneumonia and bronchitis during the first year of life in children whose parents smoke, as well as an increased frequency of admission to hospital have been observed. Children whose mothers smoke have also been found to have a higher frequency of acute bronchitis, tracheitis and laryngitis than those whose mothers are non-smokers. Acute respiratory illness during childhood may have long-term effects on the growth and development of the lungs, and might make the lungs more susceptible to the effects of active smoking, as well as to the development of chronic obstructive pulmonary disease in adult life.

- In the United States a study of 650 children aged 5–10 years showed that the prevalence of chronic wheezing was 1.9% in children whose parents were both non-smokers, 6.9% in children whose mother or father smoked, and 11.8% in children whose parents were both smokers. Children whose parents smoke have a 30–80% higher prevalence of chronic cough or phlegm than children of non-smokers, as well as an increased risk of asthma; passive smoking may also exacerbate any existing health problems (39). Asthmatic children of smokers are reported to experience improvements in their condition when their parents stop smoking (45).
- A recent study among children aged 8–11 years in Hong Kong found that parental smoking in the home was significantly associated with an increased risk of coughs and phlegm (33).

Several studies report that chronic middle ear effusions in children are related to parental smoking, being more frequent when both parents smoke.

Concurrent symptoms might appear when a child is overexposed to tobacco smoke. For example, there is a condition known as the Monday morning syndrome, which occurs when children who have been inhaling smoke during the weekend develop otitis and respiratory infections on Sunday evening and have to see

53

the doctor on Monday morning.

Another effect of passive smoking is that it predisposes and indirectly encourages children to smoke. Children of parents who smoke are more likely to smoke themselves as adolescents and adults, having been brought up in a smoking environment (see Chapter 4, p. 60).

Economic consequences

Tobacco consumption is not only a major health hazard but an economic burden on individuals and families. Economic studies in a number of developed countries have demonstrated that the costs of smoking for society are far higher than the revenue brought to the country by the tobacco industry. They include:

— The costs of direct medical care (including increased neonatal care costs).

— The cost of absenteeism from work (in Canada it has been estimated that smokers are absent from work 33–45% more than non-smokers).

— The cost of fires and industrial accidents caused by smokers and the related increased insurance costs.

— The costs related to time spent on smoking. Not only does smoking decrease the productivity of the person concerned but it may disturb non-smokers and create undue stress between workers, and between workers and employers.

— The costs related to maintenance. Smoking creates litter and necessitates more frequent renewal of decoration, furnishings and filters in ventilation systems.

The economic consequences of smoking in developing countries revolve around two main principles. Firstly, the use of tobacco increases health care costs in poor countries, where this cost is often directly borne by the individual. Secondly, many poor families spend a significant proportion of their income on tobacco instead of food. This can lead to dietary deficiencies among these families, particularly among women and young girls, who are often the last to be served at mealtimes.

  • In Bangladesh, a survey has shown that smoking five cigarettes a day in a household could lead to a monthly dietary deficit of 8000 calories; this is nearly a quarter of the monthly maintenance energy requirements of a 12-kilogram child (46).

54

The general effect of smoking is that poor families are becoming poorer, especially in rural areas, where up to 5% of monetary income may be spent on tobacco. Smoking during pregnancy adds to poverty, malnutrition, and anaemia, all of which contribute to infant death, particularly in developing countries. However, for a few countries, tobacco is also an important cash crop, and reductions in tobacco production should be compensated for by the promotion of other crops.

Some of the economic consequences of tobacco consumption may be more acutely felt by women. For example, special mention can be made of the consequences of absenteeism from work of the wage-earning partner in countries where no compensatory scheme exists; or of the consequences of children falling ill from passive smoking causing increased absenteeism from work for the person who has to take care of them.

In both developed and developing countries, the effect of the illness or death of a father will have catastrophic effects upon the life of the children and the surviving partner both psychologically and economically. If it is the mother who dies, the consequences for the children may be particularly dire.

Furthermore, in some developing countries the tobacco growing and manufacturing industries employ a substantial proportion of women. Hence, when tobacco consumption decreases, it will be necessary to consider alternative employment for these women.

Assessing further the effects of the epidemic

In developed countries the effects of smoking on women's health have been well documented. In view of their traditional social and reproductive roles, these effects may pose more risks for them than would the same behaviour in men. This greater risk should be a source of concern in all countries as smoking rates among women are increasing. There is a need for additional assessment and appreciation of the risks incurred by women compared with men. Particular care should be taken to investigate all aspects of the influence of smoking on maternal death.

In particular, there is a growing awareness of the effects of passive smoking on health but while the evidence for lung cancer is clear, further investigations are needed to clarify the role of environmental tobacco smoke in the etiology of other disease conditions and to determine the long-term consequences of passive smoking for children.

While there is now enough information to justify action, the paucity of data in many developing countries makes it a matter of urgency for studies to be conducted in these countries, to confirm the information found in other parts of the world. Section 2 of the country profile in Annex 1 gives an outline of the type of mortality and morbidity data necessary to assess the scale and effect of smoking epidemics; and section 3 provides the basic economic data necessary to analyse the economic impact of tobacco in the individual countries.

In addition to the studies described above, further socioeconomic investigations and in-depth studies are required on the relationship between smoking, family nutrition and nutritional status of women and young girls in poor countries.

A deeper understanding of the consequences of maternal illness on family life would allow a more comprehensive assessment of the wider consequences of the consumption of tobacco by women. It would also be desirable to investigate the psychological and economic effects of the death of the main carer of the family.

Chapter 4

Why women start
and continue to smoke

Many factors affect the initiation and maintenance of tobacco use by girls and women. Both internal factors such as self-esteem and self-image, as well as external factors such as social acceptability and tobacco advertising are important. Initiation factors are complex and differ, not only between developed and developing countries, but also between different groups within countries. Maintenance of consumption of tobacco is due both to nicotine dependence and to the difficulties in quitting which stem from different sociocultural backgrounds and social-structural factors such as multiple roles, low income, stress and coping behaviours.

Women are also specifically targeted by the tobacco industry through special brands, and through advertising and promotions which target their aspirations. There is also the issue that the fear of losing revenue from advertising prevents the media from reporting on the risks to women's health from smoking, to the extent warranted by the problem. Media collaboration is needed to make women aware of the hazards of smoking and help them stop. Smoking is very much a women's issue and should be recognized as such.

Smoking usually begins in adolescence, the time for discovery, challenge and experimentation, but the process of becoming a smoker may have begun in childhood.

The reasons that will motivate women to continue smoking are quite different from those pushing young girls to start. While there seems to be little gender difference in relation to why teenagers start to smoke, in some developed countries more young girls smoke than young boys. Smoking patterns vary considerably among the young from one country to another, depending on the social acceptability of tobacco, sociocultural and religious factors, the availability of tobacco, advertising, the relative cost of tobac-

57

co, and health education activities. All these aspects must be taken into consideration to understand the various stages involved in becoming a smoker, as well as the factors influencing the maintenance of smoking.

When young girls start smoking

Although some try their first cigarette as children, the majority of smokers start smoking in their teens, and most girls experiment with cigarettes around the age of 10–14 years. Girls who move from occasional to regular smoking are more likely to continue smoking into adult life. In most countries few people start smoking after the age of 18–21 years; however, in some countries such as China, prevalence is low during adolescence and increases during early adulthood.

Why young girls start smoking

The process of becoming a smoker is complex, and is intrinsically linked to social and individual motivations. Most young people try smoking for several reasons, including: stimulation and challenge (rebellion against parents or society, curiosity, excitement); to create an identity and satisfy need for self-esteem — to feel good, appear more adult and sophisticated, and look better; and to belong to a group, to be approved and accepted by friends who smoke and to avoid peer group disapproval or rejection. Many young girls also regard smoking as a way of keeping slim.

Furthermore, adolescence is often a period of rebellion and smoking is one of the risk-taking behaviours that may appeal to young girls. Smoking is often associated with alcohol and drug use as well as sexual activity in female teenagers. While these behaviours are frequently concurrent, the motivating factors can be diverse and depend on the environment.

The process of becoming a smoker essentially involves four stages: (1) awareness; (2) initiation/experimentation; (3) habituation; and (4) maintenance/dependence. These stages are influenced by sociocultural, environmental and personal factors, the influence of which is dynamic and can change over time. For some girls and women, opportunities, age or class position will affect the process of initiating and maintaining smoking.

Sociocultural factors

Social acceptability

Social acceptability refers to a situation within a specific cultural context, in which a particular behaviour is considered appropriate, so that those demonstrating the behaviour are permitted to continue, even if they are harming themselves or others. It also implies that societies may be reluctant to interfere in this behaviour.

What is particularly dangerous about tobacco is the fact that it is a legal drug which in many countries has gained a social acceptability that hitherto has gone unquestioned. Yet, in some countries, such as countries where Islam is the predominant religion, smoking by women is not socially acceptable and may even be forbidden. According to the Koran, anything that is harmful to health and to the individual, such as smoking or use of alcohol, both of which are considered destructive, should be banned. In other countries, legislation and other measures to control smoking may help to keep prevalence rates low. Smoking may, for example, be prohibited in public places, or forbidden among certain age groups, e.g. in Japan, smoking is only allowed from the age of 20. Religious and cultural beliefs may also act as a deterrent.

An overview of the estimated prevalence of smoking among women in various developing countries indicates that women are sensitive to social or religious acceptability, factors which contributed to keeping prevalence rates low among women in developed countries in the past and which are responsible for keeping rates low in most developing countries today. Care should be taken to ensure that if these social attitudes begin to disappear as these countries develop, then specific educational programmes are created so that the prevalence of smoking among women will not increase.

In the experimental stage (less than one cigarette per week), the teenager tries to create her self-image in society and this becomes reinforced with time. It is an image that she sees in others, and that is generally imposed upon her by the positive and desirable images of smoking promoted by tobacco advertising. Such images are potentially powerful influences in adolescence. The "social aspects" of smoking (e.g. use of certain brands of cigarettes), although reinforcing smoking among young smokers, become less important as the smoking behaviour develops, dependence increases and smoking becomes part of the daily routine.

Parental influence

Most children first learn about smoking from their parents, teachers or other influential figures, and are more likely to take up smoking if their parents smoke or have permissive attitudes to smoking. Learning to smoke starts with the awareness stage, where the young girl's attitude towards smoking is influenced by parents or relatives who smoke. She learns about the "dynamics" of smoking, the postures, and the places to smoke and, being a passive smoker, becomes accustomed to the smell and sight of cigarettes. In developed countries, girls in particular appear to be influenced by their parents' smoking behaviours and attitudes, although this decreases as they become older. Mothers have a particularly strong impact on their daughters' smoking behaviour, whenever they are taken as role models.

- In the United States studies have found that girls are five times more likely to take up smoking (20.3% versus 4.1%) if they live with one or both parents and an older sibling who smoke than if there are no smokers in the household (47).

- A study in New Zealand revealed that the percentage of children who had tried smoking and whose mother or father smoked was highest at 9 years of age and progressively decreased as they became older. At 9 years of age, having a friend who smoked did not influence smoking behaviour; by 11 years of age, however, it made a difference. Thirteen-year-old girls tended not to smoke if their mother was a non-smoker. Girls aged 9–15 years seemed to be influenced to try smoking if their father smoked or was an ex-smoker. Those who had never smoked by 15 years of age were likely to have a father who was a non-smoker (48).

- In Canada and the United Kingdom, studies have shown that children whose parents are smokers are twice as likely as children whose parents are non-smokers to become smokers themselves.

Parents' authority in prohibiting smoking has also been shown to play an important role in preventing early uptake of smoking.

- A study in Norway showed that 62.5% of 15-year-old students whose parents allowed them to smoke smoked daily, compared with 16.7% of students whose parents did not (12).

Peer influence

Having friends who smoke can be another predictor of future smoking. Many young people try their first cigarette because of peer influence; almost 75% of all first cigarettes are smoked with another teenager. The concept of "peer pressure" has been consistently identified as a factor influencing smoking behaviour among young people. Many young people experiment with smoking in groups, and peer approval is an important mechanism

60

for maintenance of smoking behaviour. Young people who smoke usually do so "with friends" and smoking clearly represents a sociable activity for them. Fear of rejection may lead a young girl to try a cigarette when offered one by friends whom she values. Refusal to do so might mean losing her friends who smoke, being isolated from the rest, set aside and ridiculed. On the other hand, most young people who are non-smokers have friends who do not smoke. For these reasons helping young women develop the confidence and skills to resist social pressures to smoke would contribute to a reduction in the prevalence of smoking. It is also important to show them how non-smoking can lead to an improvement in their social lives.

- An anti-smoking programme in Italy (Table 13) demonstrated that students whose best friend smokes are more likely to be smokers than are students whose best friend is a non-smoker (49).

Table 13. Concordance and discordance in smoking behaviour among friends (Italy: 562 students)

Respondent	Best friend	
	Smoker	Non-smoker
Male		
Smoker	61.8	38.2
Non-smoker	36.6	63.3
Female		
Smoker	79.7	20.3
Non-smoker	27.8	72.2

Source: reference 49.

Personal factors

Self-image

Smoking is portrayed in advertising as a means of attaining maturity, adulthood, and popularity, and of being sophisticated, sociable, feminine, and sexually attractive. In developed countries, where the media promote an image of female attractiveness which equates being thin with desirability, evidence shows that weight control and dieting are major obsessions among adolescent girls. For these girls, being slim gives them self-confidence and is fashionable.

- A Canadian study showed that two out of three teenage girls attending schools run by the London Board of Education, Ontario, were on diets by the age of 13, and 30% of them had used drastic measures such as drugs, laxatives, and vomiting while dieting. Most of these girls had also reduced their degree of participation in sports and other physical activities (*12*).

- In the United States, a survey (NIDA High School Senior Survey) showed widespread use of non-prescription diet pills among girls aged 13–18 years. Another survey showed that more smokers than non-smokers used diet pills (*47*).

Self-esteem

Studies have repeatedly found that girls who have low self-esteem are more likely to take up smoking. A recent WHO study in Europe (*50*) found that girls who felt that they had a lot of control over their health and life in general were less likely to become smokers than those who felt they had little control. Research in developed countries has shown that children who smoke are more likely to be under-achievers at school, have low academic goals, be alienated from school and be less interested in continuing with their education than children who are non-smokers.

Using smoking to bolster self-confidence stems from the widespread belief that smoking can help calm nerves, control moods and alleviate stress — all important concerns during adolescence. By showing attractive young women, with handsome male partners, socializing with groups of clearly successful and confident people, tobacco advertisements accurately evaluate young people's insecurities, and convince them that they can develop these desirable qualities if they smoke.

- A study in the United Kingdom showed that having positive beliefs about the advantages of smoking was an important predictor of taking up smoking in girls but not boys. Girls who thought that smoking made people look more grown-up, helped calm nerves and control weight, gave confidence and was enjoyable, were the most likely to start smoking (*51*).

Disposable income

For many young girls the initiation of smoking corresponds to a rise in disposable income. It has been shown, in a few countries, that teenagers may be even more sensitive than adults to the relative price of cigarettes and that the price affects not only whether teenagers smoke, but also how much they smoke. Thus a rise in the price of tobacco products can influence the level of consumption; however, even with little money, priority may be given to the purchase of cigarettes (see p. 67).

62

Knowledge

Knowledge, beliefs and attitudes about smoking also influence smoking behaviour. In developed countries, studies have shown that adolescents who smoke are usually less knowledgeable about the health risks involved, do not believe that smoking will affect them personally, or consider that the short-term benefits outweigh any health risks. However, knowledge alone is not sufficient to prevent smoking among adolescents, since many misinterpret the risks involved.

In developing countries, young girls' knowledge about smoking and its effects on health is likely to be much lower because of the lack of systematic health education programmes and the structural barriers such as scattered rural populations and high levels of illiteracy.

- In 1986, 92% of adults and 85% of smokers in the United States believed that smoking is a cause of cancer. The proportions of smokers who did not believe that smoking increases the risk of developing lung cancer, heart disease, chronic bronchitis and emphysema were 15%, 29%, 27% and 15%, respectively. These percentages correspond to between 8 million and 15 million adult smokers in the United States. Only 18% of smokers were "very concerned" about the effects of smoking on their health, and 24% were not at all concerned. About half of the smokers incorrectly believed that a person would have to smoke 10 or more cigarettes a day before health would be affected (36).

- In Finland, it was found that many smokers, while they generally accepted that smoking was harmful, thought that their consumption level was low enough not to cause any serious harm. In many studies it has been shown that most smokers, especially young smokers, believe that they will not smoke in 5 years' time, i.e. they will give up smoking in the near future (52).

- In Canada, a study of smoking behaviour among 17-year-olds found that smokers were less knowledgeable about the health risks and had more positive attitudes to smoking, were more likely to have parents and friends who smoked, were less physically attractive and in poorer physical condition, had lower levels of academic achievement, had less well-educated parents and were of lower socioeconomic status (12).

Environmental factors

Advertising and sales promotion

The tobacco industry is dependent on a mass market. Because many smokers die prematurely and others quit, the only way for the tobacco industry to maintain high levels of economic activity and profits is to recruit new smokers, especially from among women and the young. The art of marketing is to tailor a product to appeal to specific target groups after a careful analysis of the potential market within a country, by projecting its image through packaging, advertising and promotions, and adjusting whenever possible and necessary its price and availability.

The tobacco industry actively promotes the view that tobacco promotions, including advertising and sponsorship, do not increase cigarette sales or encourage people to start smoking, but merely affect the brand choice of adult smokers. There is now considerable evidence from developed countries that children are aware of tobacco advertising, that tobacco promotions influence whether young people start and continue to smoke, and that in countries that have banned cigarette advertising, cigarette smoking has declined more rapidly among young people than in countries that have not.

- Although tobacco advertising had been banned in the countries of central and eastern Europe, the recent economic changes have raised the question of allowing advertising. The transnational tobacco industry has responded by launching an extensive marketing and advertising campaign in these countries. In Hungary, for example, where tobacco advertising had been banned by a ministerial regulation (not by a law), the situation is now being reconsidered. The transnational tobacco industry has begun sales promotions by distributing patches, umbrellas, watches and similar items which tempt the local small businesses and are already visible in the streets. There are few established mechanisms and little experience in enforcing the existing regulations (personal communication, T. Piha, 1991).

- In 1986, a transnational tobacco company introduced a "female brand" of cigarettes into Hong Kong, clearly targeted at young women, with images of emancipation, slimness, beauty and desirability. Only about 1% of women under the age of 40 years smoked in Hong Kong at the time, so this was a clear attempt to create a market. It would thus seem to have little relevance to "brand-switching", which the tobacco industry frequently claims is the purpose of its advertising.

Over the past few years in developed countries and in some developing countries, the tobacco industry has targeted both its products and its advertising at women in a number of ways:

— The promotion of brands through advertisements and sponsorship using images and messages that depict smoking as being glamorous, sophisticated, romantic, sexy, healthy, sporty, relaxing, liberated, rebellious and, last but not least, slimming, although in countries where to be slim is not the fashion, this message is omitted. Cigarette companies have also portrayed smoking as a "torch of freedom", a "tool of beauty" and a sign of progress.

— Advertising in women's magazines. This not only encourages smoking by women but may also discourage reporting about the risks of smoking to women's health. In some countries, it has been shown that magazines that are dependent on revenue from cigarette advertising are less likely to cover the health hazards. This has been demonstrated by the case of a famous magazine in the USA that disclosed the details of the compromises it had been forced into before it stopped including advertisements in 1990.

- A survey (1990–91) of the most popular women's magazines in 13 European countries, which together have over 50 million female readers, found that 69% of the magazines accepted cigarette advertisements and only 22% had given major coverage to smoking and health issues in the previous year. Although the majority of these magazines refused or avoided using images of models smoking, two out of five had no restrictions on using such photographs. Indeed, some magazines, particularly those from France, Italy and Spain, appeared to be promoting smoking through the widespread use of positive images of models smoking (53).

- It has been estimated that in the United Kingdom, despite restrictions on tobacco advertising, a collective readership of 7 million women aged 15–24 years are exposed to tobacco advertising through women's magazines. Magazines that refused cigarette advertisements were more likely to have covered smoking and health issues than those that accepted cigarette advertisements. Indeed, revenue from cigarette advertising increased between 1985 and 1989, while coverage of smoking and health issues declined (53).

While a few television and radio networks and magazines now reject tobacco advertising, others attempt to justify it with arguments such as:

— readers are responsible for what they read and can make their own judgements;

— the media are not responsible for the outcome as far as cigarette advertising is concerned;

— cigarette advertisements are acceptable as long as they carry a health warning;

— the advertising policy is determined by the publishers and there is no right to impose censorship.

Other sectors of the leisure industry, such as sport and the arts have also become dependent on revenue from tobacco companies, particularly for the organization of international sporting events and the staging of expensive productions. Glamorous models, successful individuals and sporting personalities, teenage pop idols and film stars all feature in cultural events, TV soap operas, plays and films which depict smoking as being an essential component of their success. These programmes, films and magazines reach many different audiences around the world and, particularly in developing countries, may create aspirations and images of sophisticated life often equated with Western life-styles, which are both unrealistic and harmful to their audience's health.

Cigarette companies also have other ways of targeting women, such as through female sports sponsorship (e.g. tennis), support of women's organizations, and funding of other activities.

In the developing countries there are few limitations on tobacco advertising, and therefore its influence on young girls, who may have little knowledge about the harmful effects of smoking, may be even more powerful than in developed countries. At present tobacco advertising in developing countries tends to be directed at the general public, although there is evidence that women are becoming special targets. In Asia, women are considered to represent a potential market for tobacco, and evidence suggests that even where tobacco advertising is prohibited by regulations, such as in China, it is still widespread.

Product development and marketing

As public awareness of the health effects of tobacco has grown, in many countries the tobacco companies have responded by increasing the amount and variety of tobacco products and promotions that are targeted specifically at women. A common characteristic of these efforts is an attempt to pre-empt or allay health concerns by introducing cigarettes with lower tar and nicotine yields; however, these do not significantly lower the risk of many tobacco-related diseases. Indeed, people who switch to low-nicotine cigarettes often compensate for the reduction by inhaling more deeply or smoking more often.

The tobacco industry may even create "women only" brands, using particular colours, shapes, sizes, names and tastes to give women the impression that if they smoke, they will be successful, youthful, happy and healthy. This has been done in developing as well as developed countries, as exemplified by the promotion of a "female brand" in India in 1990. This marketing is often complemented by tobacco sales in places frequented by women, such as dress shops and grocery stores. This approach needs to be recognized early if it is to be properly counteracted. Another marketing strategy designed to appeal to women may be to sell the cigarettes in packages containing fewer cigarettes.

Availability

The easier tobacco is to obtain, the more likely it is that young women will use it. It is important to limit its availability to prevent dependence. As mentioned earlier, in some countries such as Japan, cultural attitudes may discourage girls from purchasing cigarettes, while in others, social or religious factors may prevent women from smoking. However, many countries do not control tobacco sales to children, and even in countries where there are laws prohibiting such sales, these are often not fully enforced and children are still able to buy cigarettes, e.g. from cigarette-vending machines.

Price

Studies in Europe and the United States have shown that the relative price of cigarettes is an important factor in determining the prevalence of smoking and tobacco consumption. Young people appear to be even more responsive to cigarette price changes than adults. Studies carried out in Austria, Finland, Ireland, the United Kingdom and the United States have shown that the demand for cigarettes varies inversely with price; when prices increase, cigarette consumption decreases. The response depends on the age and socioeconomic status of the smoker. Similarly, a study in rural Nepal has shown that saving was a major reason for stopping smoking.

In some countries it is difficult for certain groups to afford cigarettes. In Peru, for example, cigarette smoking is adopted by the more affluent and literate Peruvians and the Indian population rarely smokes because cigarettes are too expensive. Poverty may also mean limited access to television and other media advertising. In other countries, however, cigarettes are made available to low socioeconomic groups. For example, in Egypt and India, cigarettes are sold singly as well as in packs, and cheaper forms of tobacco products (bidis, hand-rolled cigarettes and hookah) mean that many people can afford to smoke.

Smoke-free environment

A smoke-free environment, in public or at home, is self-promoting. A young girl who is used to living in a smoke-free environment is likely to perceive the odour of tobacco smoke as unpleasant and later on to insist on clean air at work as well as at home, thus contributing to the concept of a tobacco-free society and life-style as the social norm.

67

Social disadvantage, assessed by measures such as parents' education and occupational level, has been shown in several developed countries to be a predictor of smoking. This may be partly because children in these countries who grow up in socially and economically disadvantaged families and communities are more likely to be exposed to smoking through their families and the community. It might also be because they have less access to other leisure and recreational pursuits as well as experiencing greater levels of alienation.

Smoke-free workplaces prevent people from starting to smoke in stressful situations, which are reported to be a cause of smoking initiation among young workers. Smoke-free public places such as restaurants are important in underlining the prevailing social norm, and also in helping smokers to quit and preventing relapse.

Smoke-free environments are particularly important in schools, where they should form part of a comprehensive policy on smoking which includes staff and students.

- A study in the United States found that the prevalence of smoking was lowest in schools that had the most comprehensive smoking policies which covered smoke-free environments as well as education on smoking (54).

Why do smokers continue to smoke?

The maintenance of smoking behaviour has been studied in many developed countries where it has been found to be influenced by a number of interrelated factors. The pressures that encourage a young girl to smoke are also important in determining whether she continues or decides to quit, and whether she is successful in doing so. As the experimenter becomes a regular smoker dependent on nicotine, a young woman's rationalization of her behaviour and dependence may be added factors in her continuing to smoke.

Some of these factors may also be valid in developing countries; however, research is required to identify which ones and to determine those that may be most prominent in the context of economic development.

Physiological factors

Dependence

Nicotine is a potent psychoactive drug (see Chapter 3). Once

68

the teenager has progressed beyond the initiation and experimental phases and her body has adapted to the effects of nicotine, smoking behaviour becomes established and dependence is created.

- A recent study in the United Kingdom has indicated that nicotine can play an active role in reinforcing smoking from a very early stage. The saliva cotinine concentration of young occasional smokers indicated that some were inhaling and obtaining pharmacologically significant doses of nicotine (55, 56).

Mild, low-nicotine cigarettes facilitate the initiation of smoking during the learning process, and as a young girl or woman begins to smoke regularly, her body gets used to regular doses of nicotine and she becomes physiologically dependent. She develops a pattern of daily smoking, such as smoking after meals and at coffee breaks. Having partners and friends who smoke reinforces the dependence.

Weight

Since many women in developed countries believe giving up smoking will lead to a weight gain (and studies have shown a weight gain of about 2–4 kg after giving up smoking among some women), they may continue to smoke in order to control their weight. Smoking becomes a way of avoiding eating, an appetite suppressant or an aid in dieting. It is well documented that smokers have a lower mean weight than ex-smokers and non-smokers. Although a variety of factors may explain this observation, there is evidence of a direct effect of smoking on metabolism. Studies in animals have shown that administration of nicotine increases metabolic rate. Furthermore, nicotine has been shown to have a greater effect on body weight and eating behaviour in female rats than in males. In humans, nicotine has been found to cause a marked increase in metabolic rate, both at rest and during light exercise.

Psychosocial factors

Psychosocial factors influencing the maintenance of smoking can be negative, such as stress and negative emotions, or positive, such as to obtain pleasure; the former seem to be the major influence in women, the latter in men.

Negative emotions

Women smokers report that smoking helps them cope with loneliness, sadness, grief, anger and frustration. It is something to hold on to when something else is lost, as it is comforting and is sometimes the only support available.

Many women find themselves under constant pressure at work and at home. The employed woman often has many roles to assume — a job to perform, a boss to please, a house to run, a family to care for — and in having to meet the demands, expectations and needs both at work and at home, she is confronted with many role conflicts. Many women smokers believe that smoking calms their nerves, relieves stress, and reduces feelings of anger and frustration. In societies where it is not acceptable to show emotions such as anger, hostility, and aggressiveness, cigarettes help restrain those negative feelings. In addition, the smoking of a cigarette gives the opportunity for a pause in a busy day.

Many women who are dependent on tobacco also believe that they cannot cope without cigarettes. Many smokers, including young smokers, experience nicotine withdrawal symptoms on quitting, such as increased craving for nicotine, irritability, restlessness and decreased concentration. Thus, rather than being a direct effect of their smoking, feeling calmer may result from relief of incipient withdrawal symptoms. The critical testing times for smokers who decide to give up are associated with negative emotions, and there is evidence that relapse is more likely to occur in such situations.

Some women may structure their day with cigarettes, using them as excuses for breaks or as rewards. Women in low-status jobs may smoke to break monotony and help them deal with frustrating tasks. Many women on low incomes, with little time to themselves, see cigarettes as their only luxury.

A young mother surrounded by children may find that the only moment of peace and relaxation, and indeed, her only treat of the day, is to light a cigarette while having a cup of coffee. Since young mothers often feel isolated from the world outside the home, they may use smoking as a way of identifying with the adult world, escaping the pressure of daily tasks, and separating themselves from their children.

Social environment

Women may smoke to maintain an image, to be accepted by others and to adhere to social conformity. The behaviour may be reinforced by the environment, such as friends who smoke, smoking areas, tobacco advertising and social pressure.

Which women smoke?

In countries with the longest history of widespread smoking, it was the more affluent and educated women who first took up smoking, but they were also the first to give it up. As described in Chapter 2, the women who are now most likely to smoke, at least in developed countries, are those on low incomes, with low-status jobs, or who are economically inactive (unemployed), are single, separated or divorced, have low levels of academic achievement, or are from underprivileged ethnic groups. Lack of education and low income may also mean less access to adequate information concerning smoking and its effects on health and less opportunity to change their way of life.

• In the United Kingdom, quantitative and qualitative research has shed light on why mothers on low incomes continue to smoke. These studies have revealed the budgeting strategies that poor households develop in the struggle to meet needs and avoid debt. Poor families give priority to essential items such as housing, fuel and food and severely restrict spending on non-essential and personal items (such as clothes, hobbies and alcohol). Consequently, minimal spending by women might be anticipated as they are usually responsible for making ends meet, particularly those in households with children where the needs of the younger generation place additional financial pressures on the adults (57). However, tobacco is one exception to the economic rule by which low-income families organize their finances. Unlike most other categories of household expenditure, spending on tobacco is inversely related to income (see Table 14).

Furthermore, spending on tobacco among low-income households with children is higher than among low-income households without children.

Table 14. Weekly expenditure of households with two adults and two children in the United Kingdom, 1988

Item of expenditure	Weekly expenditure (£)[a]			
	Household income under £175 a week		All households	
Housing	15.52	(13)	32.51	(16)
Fuel, light, power	10.08	(8)	11.41	(6)
Food	34.21	(28)	42.99	(22)
Alcohol	5.46	(4)	7.84	(4)
Tobacco	5.55	(5)	4.24	(2)
Clothing, footwear	7.40	(6)	15.92	(8)
Household goods	20.05	(16)	33.37	(17)
Transport	12.75	(10)	27.99	(14)
Services	11.59	(9)	21.56	(11)
Miscellaneous	0.68	(0.5)	1.28	(0.6)
Total	**123.29**		**199.11**	

[a] Figure in parentheses gives expenditure as a percentage of total weekly expenditure.

Source: reference 57.

The highest per capita expenditure on tobacco is among one-adult house-holds with children.

Qualitative studies of caring highlight the experiences that underlie these associations between smoking, poverty and caring for children. In one study of 57 mothers caring for children in low-income households, half were smokers. These women described how smoking was associated with breaks from caring, where they rested and had something to eat and drink. Cigarettes were not only associated with the maintenance of normal caring routines, they were part of the way women coped with breakdowns in these patterns of caring. In particular, smoking was described by smokers as a major strategy employed when their children's demands became "too much to cope with".

When asked what they did in these circumstances, the respondents typically described how they created a space — symbolic if not physical — between themselves and their children and then filled this space with a self-directed activity. Smoking a cigarette was the major self-directed activity for mothers who smoked.

In these conditions, other luxury items and leisure activities had been surrendered in the pressure to make ends meet. As other studies have found, the level of spending on clothes, shoes, make-up, haircuts and non-essential food items by these mothers was low. Within a life-style devoid of personal spending, cigarettes could be the only item that women bought for themselves (57).

Women who are subject to discrimination or oppression (such as battered women, victims of sexual assault, immigrants, racial minorities, single mothers, and women with disabilities) may be more likely to be smokers. Research is needed among these groups to develop and make available appropriate public education and public information programmes, as well as support and counselling services on tobacco control.

In countries where cigarette smoking is comparatively new among women, the fact that it has been adopted by the more affluent professional women may be due to the more liberated environment in which they live and work, their relative affluence and their urban environment which expose them to tobacco advertisements and make cigarettes more accessible. Nevertheless, it should be emphasized that in some countries, such as India, women in rural areas still use tobacco more than those in urban areas do.

Women as role models

In many occupations, women present a social and behavioural image which is taken as a role model by girls and other women.

Women, as primary carers and educators of children and others, are in a powerful position to influence smoking behaviour.

Consequently, they can play an important role in smoking prevention and cessation.

For children and adolescents, their mothers, friends and schoolteachers can all have a positive effect by encouraging them not to smoke and by setting an example. Later on, women in health professions, i.e. primary health care workers, nurses, and doctors, can also serve as educators by informing and advising patients, such as pregnant women or women on the pill. As women may prefer to go to female doctors, they may be more likely to confide in them, express their concerns, and if they smoke accept advice on quitting. Studies have shown that physician advice is particularly effective with light smokers.

Women in sport and the media can also reverse the social acceptability of smoking among women and show that those who do not smoke are healthy, attractive and beautiful, and that intelligent women do not smoke.

Women in political, governmental and nongovernmental organizations, while dealing with women's issues, are well placed to encourage women to stop smoking and can help promote non-smoking behaviour. They can also be instrumental in the passing of legislation and/or regulations.

Activists in the women's movement can also influence the image of cigarette smoking. Equating smoking to women's equality has been criticized by a number of feminist thinkers. Smoking is a feminist issue in terms of the smoking-related morbidity and mortality in women. It is also identified as a feminist issue because cigarette advertising is promoting a distorted and misleading image of smoking.

Documenting the epidemic

To determine the extent of the epidemic and to develop the means for action against the consumption of tobacco by women, not only are standardized epidemiological data necessary, but behavioural studies are needed to increase our understanding of the factors that influence smoking and smoking behaviour in different populations.

While the motivations of girls and women in developed countries have been partially documented, not enough has been done to identify the determinants of smoking for women in developing countries. An analysis of the influence of the different factors encouraging or preventing women from smoking in different economic and sociocultural settings are important subjects for health system and socioeconomic research at national and regional levels and universities should be encouraged to undertake such research. Sections 4, 5 and 6 of the country profile in Annex 1 indicate the type of information that should be collected to document the epidemic in individual countries.

While legislation against tobacco advertising is a priority, in countries where such laws have not yet been passed, research is needed on the marketing techniques used to target women and girls.

Chapter 5

Prevention and cessation of tobacco use

Prevention and cessation of smoking among women and girls require a series of measures, including public information, school health education, and restrictions on marketing, advertising and the availability of tobacco. However, most current tobacco control programmes fail to recognize and address the specific needs of women. Thus, women and girls are often not armed with the appropriate knowledge and skills to avoid starting to use tobacco or to stop. Currently, organized cessation programmes are used by only a small proportion of smokers; the majority of smokers who quit do so without the support of a formal programme, though they are influenced by information propagated through campaigns or more generally. Evaluation studies need to address both approaches to quitting. Whenever prevention programmes are developed, they should include, from the onset, components specific to tobacco consumption by women. Evaluation studies and research must cover sex-specific issues in order to develop adequate prevention and cessation programmes. The transferability of tools and techniques relevant to women is the key to their application in developing countries, where the priority is to develop programmes that are immediately affordable.

Many factors are involved in determining whether a girl starts and continues to smoke, if and when she attempts to quit, and her chances of success in quitting. The relative importance of these factors varies between individuals and populations and it is, therefore, neither possible nor appropriate to select just one or two to be addressed.

Accordingly, comprehensive action to address all the relevant factors is needed. A combination of measures, at the community, national and international levels, should be aimed at discouraging the uptake of smoking and encouraging cessation. There are already many examples of effective action, particularly in developed countries, which can be drawn on. However, there is a need to adapt these approaches to make them appropriate to the specific situation in different countries. It will also be necessary to develop new approaches in areas where current initiatives are limited or unsuccessful.

Preventing the uptake of smoking

Possibly nowhere more than in tobacco control is the saying "Prevention is better than cure" more true. However, much remains to be done to ensure that preventive measures are used effectively.

Information and health education

School health education

There have been a number of successful health education programmes; however, the health education needs of women smokers in developed countries were neglected until the mid-1980s. Even then, health education was often inappropriate for them and thus the reduction in the prevalence of smoking among girls has been less than that achieved among boys. It is essential that developing countries should not be tempted to dismiss the need for health education for women on the basis that smoking is not currently a major problem.

Health education is initially given by parents in the home, consciously or unconsciously. The next contact will be through health education programmes in schools. However, there is no universal recipe that will guarantee the success of school health education programmes on tobacco; success is heavily dependent on social, cultural and behavioural factors. The effectiveness of such programmes has varied considerably, with more positive results being observed in programmes developed towards the end of the 1970s and during the 1980s.

The programmes that have been successful in reducing smoking rates in children are those that have done more than simply provide information about the long-term health effects of smoking — which often means little to young girls and women — and have attempted to improve personal and social skills. These programmes point to some common factors for success, such as the incorporation of a "tobacco or health" component within a more

76

comprehensive approach covering other essential elements of a healthy life-style. The programmes thus aim to improve young people's knowledge about the effects of tobacco use through discussions and participatory learning methods; to develop personal and social skills to help young people resist social pressure to smoke; to involve the family, in order to reinforce the health education given in school; and to influence school authorities to provide smoke-free environments and especially, to prevent the teachers from smoking.

- Studies in Norway and the United Kingdom have demonstrated that the involvement of parents in prevention programmes can lead to significant reductions in the tobacco consumption of children and parents (50).

The age at which young girls should start to be educated about the harmful effects of tobacco consumption will depend on the country. Schools could use a "spiral curriculum" approach, i.e. the subject is taught not just once but at several different points in the child's education, in ways that are appropriate to the child's stage of development. This would involve educating children in nursery schools and elementary schools about the danger and unpleasantness of smoking before they begin to think about taking it up, and teaching them to regard non-smoking as the social norm before they reach their teens. Such a programme has been introduced in Canada, to address children aged 3–6 years. This could be followed with children aged 9–10 years, before they start to experiment with tobacco, with information on health and how to deal with social influences. This could be reinforced later with programmes aimed at maintaining non-smoking behaviour and helping children who have taken up smoking to give it up. Although many programmes have been shown to influence knowledge and attitudes to smoking, only a few have had any impact on delaying or reducing onset of smoking.

- Evaluation of an anti-smoking educational programme among Italian adolescents showed that most teenagers knew about the harmful effects of cigarette smoking, but this did not prevent them from smoking. However, the programme had some effect on occasional and light smokers (49).
- Similarly, a study of children aged 9–15 years in New Zealand showed that knowledge of health risks did not prevent them from smoking (48).
- Data from the United Kingdom revealed that both children who were smokers and those who were non-smokers knew about the harmful effects of smoking. For smokers, however, such knowledge was counterbalanced by positive perceptions related to smoking such as being part of growing up, better mood, increased confidence, and making friends more easily (58).

77

- The British Cancer Research Campaign has developed two programmes which have been successful in preventing young people from smoking. "The problems of C932" is aimed at 9- and 10-year-olds and involves parents. "The search for Dr Ricardo" is a video targeted at children of about 12 years old, who are at an age when they are likely to start smoking.

In many developed countries, school health education programmes have been effective in increasing young women's knowledge about the health effects of smoking, increasing their awareness of influences such as advertising and social pressure, and developing their self-confidence, self-esteem and social skills to resist pressure to start and continue smoking. Since girls often believe that smoking helps them deal with stressful situations, many educators consider that developing girls' self-esteem and competence to solve problems themselves is the most appropriate and effective way of enabling them to cope with life without resorting to smoking.

School health education has limitations, however, arising from the amount of time students may be exposed to negative influences through contact with peers, family, and the media compared with the little time spent on health education. In many developed countries it has been found that young people who become regular smokers are more likely to be alienated from school, and are therefore unlikely to be reached or influenced by school health education programmes. In addition, in developing countries many young girls do not attend school. It is therefore important that programmes are developed that use other youth and educational networks such as youth clubs, religious organizations and sports organizations, particularly as they adopt less didactic approaches.

Public information

Most public information programmes have not been sufficiently sex-specific; they have not been targeted at young girls. Messages on smoking and health can be communicated through several channels, selected for their appeal to women and adapted to the needs of those in developed and developing countries. The objectives of such public information programmes are:

— to increase women's awareness of the hazards of smoking;

— to increase awareness among decision-makers of the need for smoking control and of the possibilities for action;

— to control the smoking epidemic and the specific dangers for women;

— to provide motivation and support for women who want to quit;

— to counteract the effects of inaccurate information and advertising.

Several factors should be considered when using different forms of media, such as the characteristics of the target audience (including the level of literacy), accessibility of information, geographical location and cultural background. Each of the media has its own specific characteristics, which should be understood and exploited. The messages should use positive language to describe the desired behaviour and to counteract the messages communicated through tobacco advertising.

Radio and television: can reach large audiences, especially through programmes popular with women; can provide examples and promote non-smoking as a healthy and attractive life-style; and can reach illiterate populations.

Newspapers and magazines: information on the effects of tobacco consumption and different ways of quitting should be included in women's magazines and journals which, through careful selection, can be used to reach women from different age groups and different social and cultural backgrounds.

Posters, billboards, and pamphlets: can provide visual examples and information to support non-smoking; can be used to reach specific target groups such as pregnant women, adolescents, etc.

Cinema: short films on non-smoking could be run before the main feature, but the first priority is to reduce or eliminate the portrayal of smoking in the films produced, a comment which also applies to television productions.

Puppet shows and presentations: these have proved successful, particularly in rural areas and villages, as they are entertaining and direct.

Promoting a tobacco-free image

In countries where the socially accepted image for a woman is already that of a non-smoker or a non-chewer of tobacco, the issue will be to maintain this attitude as these societies pass through phases of female emancipation and economic development. In other countries, ways should be found to promote this healthy image, emphasizing positive aspects such as attractiveness, glamour and liberation and to make non-smoking look healthy, socially attractive and emancipated. In addition, women should be made aware of the special health risks related to reproduction.

- A national media campaign aimed at young women and using television, cinema and women's magazines has been developed in Australia. One of the main themes is that you do not need to smoke to enjoy yourself.

Restrictions on the availability of tobacco

Legislation restricting the availability of tobacco can be an effective instrument to reduce smoking, particularly if accompanied by appropriate health education. For a number of years, WHO has been promoting several measures to control smoking, some of which may be more effective for women.

Control of advertising and sales promotion

The influence of tobacco advertising and other sales promotions on women has been described in Chapter 4. Legislation restricting or prohibiting media advertising (television, radio, cinema, poster and press), distribution of free samples, sponsorship of sports and cultural events, special discount schemes, as well as other direct and indirect advertising strategies, can greatly reduce the desire of women to smoke.

Taxation

Price increases can help reduce tobacco sales, especially among young people and women, who often have little personal income to spend on themselves. Studies in a number of developing countries have found that, on average, a 1% increase in the real price of cigarettes leads to a 0.5% decrease in consumption among adults and even more among young people; the reduction may be even greater in developing countries. However, there are valid reasons for careful consideration of every proposed increase in tobacco duty. For those on low incomes, unable to reduce their consumption, a price increase can simply create a downward spiral: as the burden of financial pressure gets heavier, the need to smoke increases with further detrimental consequences to health as the quality of life deteriorates. One way of solving this dilemma is for governments to create ways in which increased tax revenues could be invested in health promotion activities, as occurs in Australia, Finland, Iceland and the United States (California). Increased welfare benefits to offset the adverse effects of price increases could also be provided.

Sales restrictions

Sales restrictions, if properly enforced and ideally preceded by health education, may have some influence on the consumption of tobacco by young girls.

A number of measures can be taken to control the illegal sale of tobacco to minors:

— a minimum age (18–21 years) should be adopted for the sale of tobacco;

— fines for selling tobacco to minors should be increased;

— tobacco access laws should be rigorously enforced;

— vendors should be required to make it clear (through warning signs in the stores) that tobacco will not be sold to minors;

— cigarette-vending machines should be eliminated;

— national campaigns should be launched regularly to inform parents, health professionals and other community organizations about the problem.

• A study in California, USA, showed that an education campaign involving the community and vendors, combined with a broad-based media campaign, reduced tobacco sales to minors. Following a six-month campaign, the over-the-counter sales of cigarettes were reduced from 74% to 39%, although sales from vending machines were not reduced (59).

Health warnings

It is imperative that the specific risks of smoking to women should always be included in health warnings on cigarette packets and advertisements, as is the case now in numerous countries, such as Canada, Iceland and Sweden. Since 1970, WHO has recommended that cigarette packets should carry health warnings in order to inform smokers about the dangers of smoking; these warnings must be accurate and comprehensible to the public, they should be changed regularly to ensure that smokers do not become accustomed to the same message and they should be clearly visible.

Other measures

Information about the potentially hazardous constituents of

tobacco on cigarette packets and restrictions on smoking in public places and in the workplace deter both women and men from smoking. Several studies have found that restrictions on smoking in the workplace lead to an overall reduction in consumption among smokers which is not made up for by increased smoking outside work. However, women in certain occupations may be exposed more specifically to environmental tobacco smoke, e.g. flight attendants and waitresses.

New forms of tobacco products should be banned to stop the tobacco industry's move to interest young non-smokers in different products.

Cessation of tobacco use

Until recently, most of the studies on quitting reported in the literature concentrated on developed countries, where tobacco use was already widespread. There have, however, been a number of successful cessation programmes in the Indian subcontinent. As tobacco use is now becoming more popular among women in developing countries, the issue is becoming increasingly important there.

The vast majority of people who stop smoking (up to 90%) do so on their own, after being influenced by a number of factors. However, smoking among women cannot be dissociated from personal, social and economic factors, which are all interrelated.

Many women want to give up smoking for a number of reasons, such as: freedom from dependence on tobacco, health, pregnancy and financial worries. However, once women start smoking, they may find it more difficult to quit than men because of a lack of social support, more reliance on cigarettes to cope with stress and anxiety, and fear of weight gain. In order to give up smoking, women need help and support to overcome the short-term physiological withdrawal symptoms that may occur when smoking is discontinued and to break behavioural patterns that may have developed over many years. They may need to talk to others and get their advice and opinions before changing their behaviour or dealing with problems in general. Hence, when designing cessation programmes, all these aspects need to be taken into account.

Some reports from organized cessation programmes have indicated that women are less successful than men in quitting. Since women in Australia, the United Kingdom and the United States are now giving up smoking at about the same rate as men, this conclusion would seem to be incorrect; however, these figures do not show the relative success of women and men in maintaining their non-smoking. The differences in cessation rates between different groups of women are, however, indisputable. Disadvantaged women who live in particularly difficult circumstances are less likely to give up smoking than better-off middle-class women.

Although many women manage to refrain from smoking for a long time, they may relapse in situations involving negative emotions, such as conflicts, stress or loss. Men, however, tend to relapse in positive situations, such as at social events. Women are less likely to relapse if they have social support, especially from friends, family and partners.

The benefits of smoking cessation

The 1990 report of the US Surgeon-General (60) is dedicated to the health benefits of smoking cessation; its major conclusions, applying both to women and men, are summarized below:

- Smoking cessation has major and immediate health benefits for women and men of all ages. These benefits apply to people with and without smoking-related diseases.

- Ex-smokers live longer than continuing smokers. For example, women who quit smoking before the age of 50 have half the risk of dying in the next 15 years compared with those who continue to smoke.

- Smoking cessation decreases the risk of lung cancer, other cancers, myocardial infarction, stroke, and chronic obstructive pulmonary disease; however, smoking cessation has more immediate effects on cardiovascular diseases than on lung cancer or chronic obstructive pulmonary disease.

- The health benefits of smoking cessation far exceed any risks from the average weight gain (2.3 kg) or any adverse psychological effects that may follow quitting.

- Women who stop smoking before pregnancy or during the first 3–4 months of pregnancy reduce their risk of having a low-birth-weight baby relative to that of women who are non-smokers: however, evidence from two intervention trials suggests that reducing daily cigarette consumption without quitting has little or no effect on birth weight.

In addition, the report underlines some specific advantages for pregnant women: those who stop smoking at any time up to the 30th week of gestation have infants with a higher birth weight than do women who smoke throughout pregnancy. Recent estimates of the prevalence of smoking during pregnancy, combined

with an estimate of the relative risk of low birth weight in smokers, suggest that 17–26% of low-birth-weight births could be
prevented by eliminating smoking during pregnancy. In groups
with a high prevalence of smoking (e.g. women with less than a
high school education), this figure could be as high as 29–42%.

- In the United States, approximately 30% of women who are cigarette
  smokers quit when they become pregnant, with greater proportions quitting among married women and especially among women with higher
  levels of educational attainment (*60*).

In societies where being thin is considered aesthetically
desirable, the fear of putting on weight has discouraged many
women from trying to give up smoking and has precipitated
relapse among many of those who had given up. An investigation
concluded that the average weight gain after smoking cessation
(2.3 kg) posed a minimal health risk. Approximately 80% of
smokers who quit gain weight and women gain more weight than
men. However, the average weight of smokers after cessation is no
greater than the weight of non-smokers. This strongly suggests
that nicotine causes artificial and reversible weight loss, which is
greater in women than men. Nevertheless, there is tremendous individual variation in the metabolic response to smoking and smoking cessation.

Quitting techniques

Stopping smoking and tobacco consumption requires an
awareness of the reasons for smoking or chewing tobacco, and
development of other ways of coping with the needs. Cessation
programmes must consider gender differences in terms of the
specific health effects of smoking, and the different needs that
women may have.

Although specific techniques can be beneficial, education is
needed to increase women's motivation to quit. Women who
smoke need to be informed about the physical and psychological
reactions involved in giving up. Girls and women who smoke
should be made aware of the positive consequences of quitting: an
improved economic situation, an improved sense of smell and
taste, more stamina, a feeling of achievement, freedom from dependence, more control over their life, and better health. Most important of all is the knowledge that it is possible to become a
non-smoker.

Quitting independently

There are many ways in which women quit on their own;
these have been popularized in various booklets and pamphlets

84

produced as guides for the general public by governmental or non-governmental organizations involved in tobacco control. Quitting independently does not mean women are giving up smoking without help, as their decision may often be the result of information and education campaigns and other forms of assistance. For example, the World No-Tobacco Days serve, once a year, to publicize the ill-effects of tobacco consumption and encourage tobacco users to stop for one day in the hope that they will continue to abstain.

General techniques

The craving for tobacco is maintained by pharmacological, social, and psychological determinants, all of which need to be considered in breaking nicotine dependence.

A number of techniques are available for both women and men. Tobacco dependence can be broken in several ways:

- *Pharmacological treatments*: e.g. nicotine replacement strategies, in which the smoker is given an alternative substance which provides temporary relief from the signs and symptoms of tobacco withdrawal; and nonspecific pharmacotherapy, in which the patient is treated symptomatically. However, specific guidance needs to be given to pregnant women.

- *Behavioural treatments*: e.g. aversive strategies to cigarette smoke (distaste, disgust, fear or displeasure); relaxation training; "contingency contracting" (a system of reward/punishment); social support; training in problem-solving skills; stimulus control (eliminating situations in which the person is likely to smoke); programmes including a number of these strategies and support groups.

- *Other treatments*: e.g. hypnosis and acupuncture.

Specific approaches for women

While all the above-mentioned approaches may be valid for women as well as for men, a growing number of smoking cessation programmes cater specifically for women's needs. They usually include basic health education; discussion of withdrawal symptoms; strategies to maintain non-smoking and prevent relapse; continuing group support; stress management; and advice on weight management, nutrition, fitness and exercise. However, approaches stressing freedom and control over one's life may be

85

unrealistic for women who suffer from poverty, violence, stress and discrimination, as other aspects of their lives will need to be changed as well (see p. 88).

Some specific tips to help women give up smoking are given below.

Quitting tips for women

- If you smoke to distance yourself from others who depend on you (children, elderly relatives, partners, friends, etc.), try to find another way of doing this.

- If you smoke to control your emotions, experiment with other methods of releasing your feelings: e.g. writing down your thoughts, discussing issues with the people in your life, meditation or exercise.

- Try to enlist support for quitting smoking from your partner, family and friends, particularly during the first few weeks as you break your dependence on nicotine.

- Get someone to look after your children, or to relieve you of other responsibilities, even for a few hours, as you begin to learn to live without tobacco.

- Plan what you will eat and drink when you decide to quit, as opposed to concentrating on what you cannot eat. This way, you can control your food intake, and control your weight.

- Consider giving up alcohol and coffee for the first month or so, as these often serve as "triggers" for social smoking.

- Change your daily routine for a while to avoid the situations where you would normally smoke, and incorporate exercise into your life instead of smoking. This will not only make you feel better, but will prevent some weight gain as well.

- Make your immediate environment smoke-free, and remove all cigarettes and other tobacco products from your home. Ask others not to smoke in your presence during the first few weeks of quitting.

- If you relapse, and have a cigarette, do not lose confidence in your ability to quit. Consider it a learning experience, and remain committed to stopping smoking.

It has been found that women-only cessation programmes allow better dissemination of women-specific messages. These specific programmes should have a comprehensive, process-oriented approach, with the following characteristics:

Accessibility: the messages should be appropriate for all women (e.g. using tapes, films, braille, sign language, non-printed materials, etc.). Programmes must be sensitive to factors such as race, ethnicity, culture, age, and socioeconomic status.

Comprehensiveness: issues cannot be restricted to smoking behaviour only but must be placed within the context of women's experiences.

Skill-building: skills in assertiveness, identifying external and internal motivations, resisting pressure, stress management and positive health behaviour must be developed.

Support: social support, respect, acceptance and trust are most important.

- In Canada, several woman-specific cessation programmes have shown some successes. They minimize the importance of cessation and examine the woman's smoking behaviour within the context of her overall life-style. Efforts are made to identify social and political influences on smoking behaviour, as well as to increase women's understanding of why they smoke (61). The women who are most successful in quitting are those who are ready to make changes in their lives: thus, part of the programme is to encourage women to learn to take control of their health and life (12).

As most smokers who give up smoking go through a process that involves contemplation of change, action, maintenance and relapse, cessation programmes must address all stages of the process. Relapse is often perceived as a failure, but in fact is part of the learning process of cessation. Repeated relapse is to be expected in smokers who are heavily dependent on tobacco and they therefore need to be encouraged to continue trying until they succeed.

Relieving social pressure

Individual programmes should be backed up by measures aimed at changing the social and environmental factors that make giving up easier and cater for the needs of non-smokers. This would include actions as diverse as economic development or changes in the social environment, as well as increased provision of smoke-free environments and action to increase awareness of the effects of passive smoking.

Smokers who quit with support from their family and friends are more likely to maintain their non-smoking behaviour. Therefore, family members and work colleagues can be given practical suggestions to help and support the participant as she becomes a non-smoker.

If women in difficult circumstances are to be helped to take control of their lives, it is necessary to adopt strategies that address not only their smoking but also the social and economic circumstances that maintain their dependence on tobacco (such as violence against women, unequal pay, etc.). Accordingly, cessation programmes for these women must be accompanied by policies and actions to reduce inequalities.

Role of health professionals

In tobacco consumption, prevention and cessation, some groups of individuals may have an exemplary role to play (see Chapter 4, p. 72). Health professionals, such as nurses, midwives, physicians, nutritionists and others, may have a particular influence on tobacco use by girls and women. This highlights the importance of specific training in this field and the need for their awareness of their part as role models for patients. Furthermore, health workers who are non-smokers are more likely to give advice about the hazards of smoking to their patients and help them quit.

Family physicians are generally in a good position to give advice and can have a positive influence. Although most physicians believe that it is their responsibility to encourage smokers to give up smoking, many do not do so routinely.

> • In the United States, population surveys show that most adult smokers have never been advised to quit smoking by a physician. According to previous studies, physicians who are cigarette smokers are less likely to give advice on smoking than are those who are non-smokers. They are also more pessimistic concerning their patients quitting. Although physicians seem to advise those thought to be at risk and those who are already motivated (62), studies have shown that advice to quit smoking by a physician is mainly effective with light smokers (63).

Too often medical practitioners assume that their women patients are already aware of the risks associated with smoking and do not attempt to influence their attitudes and behaviour when issues related to health and life-style are addressed in medical consultations.

> • For example, a Swedish study showed that smoking was discussed in 75% of medical consultations and alcohol consumption in 30%. Whereas all men were questioned about their smoking, only half of the women were. The results also showed that the information exchanged was superficial and did not give a full picture of the patients' behaviour, except in a few cases (64).

However, some doctors, such as gynaecologists and obstetricians, may have more influence on women, because of their close relationship with the patient and their frequent contact during certain important periods of her life. Women are often highly receptive to anti-smoking education during these consultations. Prenatal care provides a good opportunity to educate women on the hazards of smoking, helping them to take control of their health and the health of their babies. More generally obstetricians and gynaecologists can advise their women patients to give up smoking when they deal with obstetric care, family planning and pregnancy, and can display and make available literature on tobacco control. Care should be taken that the approach adopted does not "blame the victim".

Paediatricians can advise parents to stop smoking when they bring in their children for consultations. The best times to talk to parents about quitting are during check-ups and visits for respiratory problems. Paediatricians may be faced with additional obstacles; for example, parents may not expect advice and may not react favourably; advice to stop smoking may not seem appropriate, especially if the child does not appear to be ill or affected by smoking.

Reasons why doctors in general fail to give advice on quitting have been identified in developed countries as: belief that it is not worth while and that the patient does not want to give up smoking; a tendency to counsel those with tobacco-related conditions, rather than light or average smokers; past failures, when advice was not followed; a feeling that providing advice is not their role; lack of confidence; feeling inadequately prepared to help; wishing to avoid embarrassing or offending the patient or discouraging her from coming back; lack of time or payment; and being unaware that simple advice can be effective. Furthermore, in developing countries, information on quitting may not be readily available.

Nurses can also encourage women to refrain from tobacco consumption, not only because nursing is still a predominantly female profession, but mainly because nurses are often in a position to give public health advice and to have contact with girls and women. To do so effectively, in many countries, the nursing profession should first address the question of nurses' own smoking.

As women may gain weight when they quit smoking, nutritionists and dieticians can provide advice on post-cessation weight management and diet as well as general advice on fitness and exercise.

Dental hygienists have a traditional role in terms of health education, where the need for good oral hygiene practices can lead to advice against tobacco consumption. The hygienist can also ask his or her patients about their use of smokeless tobacco, teach

89

them techniques for oral self-examination, detect signs of oral lesions due to smokeless tobacco products, and discourage patients from using these products.

It is evident, therefore, that health services should be tobacco-free. Smoking or use of other forms of tobacco should not be permitted in hospitals, health centres, screening facilities, ambulances, primary health care centres, pharmacies or opticians' offices, etc.

- A smoking control policy implemented in a hospital in Barcelona, Spain, over a 3-year period resulted in a reduction in smoking among hospital staff and a greater awareness of the exemplary role health professionals can have. This indicates that carefully designed programmes can be successful even in countries with high rates of smoking (65).

Halting the epidemic

Special education and cessation programmes aimed at adolescents and women have been developed in a few countries with a certain amount of success. Research needs to be carried out on an ad hoc basis to investigate which components of these programmes can be transferred to different countries and which must be modified to fit different cultures and socioeconomic backgrounds. A key to the success of these efforts is the evaluation of education programmes; in particular, school-based tobacco control education programmes need to be evaluated for their effects on girls. This will facilitate the design of corresponding tobacco control methods appropriate for girls, in various educational settings.

Programmes must also address the problem of how to reach girls and women in other settings, e.g. girls who do not attend school, women in the workplace, community centres, etc. Smoking behaviour may be easier to change with specific life events, such as marriage, pregnancy, birth of a child, divorce, change of job, etc. Are these opportunities systematically exploited in tobacco control campaigns aimed at women? Where resources are very scarce, methods should also be developed to identify high-risk groups (e.g. adolescents, young women intending to start a family, or women in certain occupations), which should be targeted for a more focused planning of smoking prevention, education and treatment.

Simultaneously, decision-makers and women themselves need to be made aware that the issue is crucial and that something can be done about it.

An important measure is the appropriate and timely training of teachers and health personnel in the prevention of tobacco use and in cessation. This cannot be done on an ad hoc basis. The appropriate skills will need to be taught through formal training included in the basic and post-basic curricula. Tobacco consumption by women is a growing problem and deserves to be treated as such in medical and public health training. Sections 6 and 7 of the attached country profile (Annex 1) can be used to monitor the actions taken at the country level to halt the epidemic.

Chapter 6

Women against tobacco: a strategy for individual, community, national and international action

The previous chapters have shown the need for urgent action to prevent the prevalence of smoking among women in developing countries from reaching the peaks that have been observed in developed countries. The previous chapters have also identified the information required to facilitate appropriate action to combat the epidemic. The tasks for all the strategists concerned are now well defined with a key role to be played by governments at all levels strengthened by international organizations, in particular WHO, nongovernmental organizations and others. These strategists will need a range of tools, including financial resources, to make them as efficient and effective as possible.

A worldwide strategy

As men in developed countries were the first to smoke in large numbers, not surprisingly researchers and policy makers first looked at these male populations to explore and, later, to counteract the effects of smoking. The previous chapters have shown the consequent imbalance in our knowledge of the smoking epidemic. These chapters have attempted to paint a picture, as yet unfinished, of the use of tobacco among women throughout the world, showing the differences between the situation in most developed countries where women smoke nearly as much as men, and the situation in developing countries where the prevalence of smoking among women is generally still low.

In view of the current situation, some universally valid actions need to be taken immediately, such as the enactment of legislation comprising all necessary measures to discourage women from using tobacco, including the provision of smoke-free places and bans on tobacco advertising. In addition, actions will have to be adapted to the specific circumstances in each country — on the one hand preventing the uptake of smoking and on the other helping smokers to quit.

A number of specific recommendations have been made at the end of each of the previous chapters; in addition, a strategy for preventing the morbidity and mortality from tobacco-related diseases in women from reaching the levels observed in men needs to be designed and applied immediately in all countries, which takes into account their different sociocultural and economic backgrounds.

This common strategy will have the following ruling objectives:

— to ensure that the "tobacco or health" situation for women is widely recognized and understood (see p. 98);

— to ensure that national control programmes are developed that contain all the measures recommended in this monograph;

— to ensure that legislation is adopted which comprises all the necessary measures to discourage women from using tobacco (such as a ban on tobacco advertising and on all other forms of promotion);

— to ensure that within the framework of national tobacco or health coordinating committees, each country secures the presence of a focal point dealing with women and tobacco;

— to ensure that school health education comprises the necessary specific tobacco control measures for girls and that public education campaigns are properly targeted at women;

— to take measures to encourage all media to provide appropriate information on tobacco or health to women of all ages;

— to take measures to empower women at all political and technical levels to develop the necessary advocatory and scientific skills to monitor and control the tobacco epidemic in women;

— to address the social and economic factors that could discourage the use of tobacco by women.

Implementing this strategy will require a strengthening of all the sectors involved to enable them to coordinate their efforts at the international, national and community levels; it will also improve knowledge of the current situation and the various tools for tobacco control.

94

Identify and strengthen the strategists

At the local, national and international levels, smoking control policies, legislation and activities are usually aimed at smokers *per se*, and the failure to take action or adopt different approaches for men and women has often been to the disadvantage of women. To redress the balance, further action needs to be taken to control tobacco use among women. To do this, the strategists concerned will need greater support. There is also a growing recognition that more of the strategists should be women.

A large number of governments and governmental organizations throughout the world have already taken effective action in tobacco control, whether by enacting legislation or adopting other measures such as supporting health education. The protection and promotion of healthy life-styles, an essential part of the health policy of certain countries, also contribute to controlling the use of tobacco. National health strategies for the prevention and control of certain diseases, such as cancer and cardiovascular disease, have usually included a strong tobacco control component and offered most of the opportunities for tobacco control. Through the establishment of health policies, governments may have the key role in controlling the tobacco epidemic in women; however, they will often need a grouping of forces behind them to motivate their action, to support it and to participate in its implementation.

The nongovernmental organizations involved in tobacco control strategies have played an important role worldwide in influencing the passing of legislation, health education and the dissemination of information. Major national and international nongovernmental organizations concerned with tobacco control should dedicate part of their programmes for the specific benefit of women.

Nongovernmental organizations dealing with women's issues have often taken little part in tobacco control efforts at global, national or community levels; although this situation is slowly changing, the mobilization of the women's movement (and women's health movement) in tobacco control also needs to be encouraged.

Community groups that can have an influence on tobacco use among women, such as parent-teacher associations, community development associations and sports organizations, should be encouraged to address the issue as a priority. The challenge involves convincing community groups not currently involved in tobacco control to apply resources to the issue of smoking and women. Of prime interest are community groups concerned with women's health or with related issues, such as occupational health and safety or environmental matters, and associations and

95

organizations concerned with particular target groups such as battered women or ethnic minorities, and particular occupational associations.

Specific community actions need to be documented and the results widely circulated. Even strong governmental action through legislation or health education will have less effect if the immediate social environment of the female smoker's workplace or community is not also conducive to quitting. Community projects should incorporate educational approaches that develop women's self-esteem and independence, and help to eliminate their need for tobacco. Attention should be given to the development and evaluation of effective weight control programmes for women who give up smoking and to their application at the community level. Public information programmes should emphasize the rights of non-smokers, especially children and pregnant women.

Occupational health programmes in factories or other places of work can be a good entry point for action and could include information on the hazards of tobacco consumption and skills-training on how to live without tobacco. The presence of health and safety committees in workplaces could facilitate the implementation of such programmes.

Specific mention should be made of the health professionals. Action by physicians, nurses and other primary health care workers has been shown to play a positive role in promoting better health for women through modification of a variety of behavioural risk factors. Such workers could be instrumental in promoting health for women by influencing their patients' behaviour and providing information. In creating a tobacco-free society, the leadership of health professionals should be mobilized through their various professional bodies and by approaching them individually; specific training should be envisaged to this effect.

The challenges facing the development of a broader-based community response to the issue of smoking among women are considerable; however, experience with raising awareness of other social and environmental issues shows that once there is widespread community concern over an issue, accelerated positive change will occur. Cooperation between all those concerned will strengthen activities by creating massive support as well as maximizing the use of limited resources.

Leaders are essential to trigger action by all the above strategists. These leaders can come from all professions: e.g. lawyers, politicians or technical specialists.

Since 1974, several WHO Expert Committees (66, 67, 68) and the WHO Study Group on Smokeless Tobacco Control (69) have made a number of recommendations for national and international action to attain, in individual countries, societies where the social norm is to abstain from tobacco consumption. Several of these recommendations specifically target national action in favour of women such as:

- recognition of the gender difference in dealing with the issue of tobacco use among women.

- legislation banning the promotion and advertising of all tobacco products; revision of legislation regarding the sale of tobacco to minors to include stiffer penalties; development of public awareness programmes among retailers to inform them of legislation regarding sales to minors; and legislation banning tobacco sales through vending machines, in order to limit accessibility to children.

- pricing policies that maintain the cost of tobacco at a high level.

- determination of the special factors influencing women to consume tobacco and health education (from primary school onwards) based on these factors; public information campaigns based on pretested strategies aimed at the specific factors in each national setting that are characteristic of female smokers.

Since 1980, World Health Assembly resolutions have mentioned the need to consider the particular health issues related to women's use of tobacco; two resolutions deserve particular attention. Resolutions WHA39.14 and WHA43.16, respectively, urge Member States to implement a nine-point smoking control strategy and to promote legislation for "progressive restrictions and concerted actions to eliminate eventually all direct and indirect advertising, promotion and sponsorship concerning tobacco".

WHO's essential role is to support the development of national tobacco control programmes at the request of its Member States. It has also developed strategies for joint action between Member States, an example of which is the European Action Plan on Tobacco for a Smoke-free Europe. The process was started at the First European Conference on Tobacco Policy in 1988, where the continent's foremost experts issued a charter against tobacco and outlined ten strategies for a smoke-free Europe. The basic principles of the charter are: that air free from tobacco smoke is an integral part of the individual's right to a healthy and unpolluted environment; that young people should be free to grow up without being subjected to undue pressure to take up smoking; that those willing to give up smoking should receive help; and that all citizens have a right to be informed of the health risks associated with smoking.

To contribute to the achievement of the worldwide objectives, WHO will, within this framework:

— ensure that data on tobacco use and related problems collected in its data centre/clearinghouse give equal coverage to women and men;

— promote and encourage and, whenever possible, support studies aimed at improving knowledge about women and smoking issues;

— ensure that its educational and public information material gives an equal emphasis to women and men.

WHO has endeavoured to sensitize the United Nations system to the harmful effects of tobacco use and obtain its support in dealing with the health, social and economic problems caused by tobacco consumption, and substantial progress has already been made in making organizations of the United Nations system tobacco-free. WHO now aims to ensure that there is a consensus on an international strategy for the whole United Nations system to disseminate information to increase awareness of the health risks of smoking, to help women avoid taking up smoking despite the influence of advertising, and to help them to quit.

The scientific integrity of WHO, its coordinating capacity, technical resources and capacity to stimulate the acquisition of new knowledge make WHO a prime mover in strengthening all strategists. It is no coincidence that some of the successes in the passing of legislation, the winning of court cases and the lowering of tobacco consumption are a result of the combined action of governments and nongovernmental organizations supported, either directly or indirectly, by WHO. Conversely, requests from governments to WHO for technical cooperation are more likely to come as a result of campaigns organized by nongovernmental organizations.

Improve knowledge

In monitoring and controlling the tobacco epidemic among women, further qualitative and quantitative research studies are important in order to identify the directions in which action should be taken. As more becomes known, new avenues will probably open for research to refine knowledge and make actions more specific and effective.

Patterns and trends of smoking among women are well documented in only a small number of highly developed countries; few developing countries have comprehensive data on the subject. A first step will be to ensure that, in countries with a well developed system of health information and statistics, data on smoking patterns and trends for women are collected and kept up to date, together with data on tobacco-related diseases. In other countries, including a large number of developing countries, rapid assessment or small-scale surveys should be carried out at regular intervals on representative samples of the population. If the expertise is not available locally or the subject is not considered a priority, the possibility of obtaining information through other health surveys should be investigated. In all cases, scientific accuracy should be emphasized, together with the necessity to collect sex-specific data. The twinning of programmes to evaluate tobacco use between developed and developing countries should be encouraged as a means of technology transfer.

Improving knowledge also means ensuring that the results of studies are comprehensible to all those who will have to take action; these data should be published and widely disseminated. As a minimum, information on the prevalence of tobacco use (percentage of women who are regular smokers or regular users of other forms of tobacco) by age group is required. The importance of age-specific information should not be underestimated. In most countries, the prevalence of cigarette smoking is significantly higher among younger women, which has important implications for prevention. Data on cigarette consumption (number of cigarettes per day), duration of exposure (age of initiation and length of time since taking up smoking), cessation rates and average tar and nicotine content of cigarettes consumed should also be obtained if possible. In countries where tobacco chewing is common among women, the prevalence of chewing and the daily consumption should also be ascertained.

There is sufficient evidence on the harmful effects of smoking to justify concerted action in all countries. While the added risks for women have also been well documented in some countries, complementary surveys could clarify the cumulative effects of ill health and poor nutrition with tobacco consumption in women in individual developing countries or in underprivileged women in other countries. Thus, further epidemiological studies are needed to improve knowledge of the health risks for women, based on samples of populations at different levels of development. Further studies are also needed to evaluate more precisely the risks of passive smoking for women, especially during pregnancy. Local and national health studies can also be effectively used to publicize the harmful effects of tobacco consumption.

Smoking and use of other forms of tobacco by women need to be understood within the context of social, cultural and behavioural influences in different populations and in different strata of the various populations. While there has recently been an increase in qualitative research on women and smoking, especially in countries where the tobacco epidemic is already affecting women, smoking as a functional behaviour needs to be analysed in relation to occupation and life circumstances, to understand why women start and continue to smoke. For example, smoking behaviours of various ethnic minorities in Canada and New Zealand have been well documented; however, little is known on the subject for most of Asia or for the general population in Africa. Similar studies will be needed to determine whether the tendency is for more girls than boys to take up smoking as countries become more economically developed.

The role of smoking in women's daily lives in developed and developing countries needs to be more fully examined, in particular regarding maintenance of smoking behaviour. Better understanding of smoking patterns among the socially disadvantaged (women on low incomes, unemployed women, battered women, women belonging to minority groups) should facilitate research into alternative coping methods appropriate to different life circumstances, and control within the working environment. It is also important to understand motivation to smoke at an individual level, as well as the links between women's experiences and smoking.

Behavioural research could also cast new light on the initiation of smoking in young people. In developing countries where the prevalence of smoking among women is still very low, the factors responsible for this situation should be carefully studied with a view to maintaining it as these societies go through phases of female emancipation and economic development. The stabilizing factors for young people and adolescents should also be assessed in various sociocultural backgrounds and educational programmes developed to help parents influence their children (primary school age) and to promote the influence of leaders and role models on adolescents.

While legislation against tobacco advertising and other forms of promotion is a priority, in countries where such laws have not yet been passed, research is needed on cost-effective methods to counter tobacco advertising and to develop effective messages to promote prevention and cessation. Such studies will increase the recognition of the importance of gender differences in the physiology and social psychology of smoking, as well as more fully reflect women's own experiences and interpretations of their smoking behaviour in dealing with prevention and cessation.

100

In view of the urgency with which tobacco control programmes need to be implemented in developing countries, in a way and at a cost they can afford, studies are required on the cost-effectiveness of various interventions to promote non-smoking, with emphasis on mass media approaches and methods to counter tobacco advertising.

Throughout the world, the effects of national tobacco control policies on smoking trends among women need to be analysed. Case-studies of activities to promote non-smoking and of tobacco control policy interventions from process and managerial points of view, would facilitate the further development of specific action for women.

However, the need for further studies and research should not delay the implementation of available strategies to control tobacco use among women.

Provide the tools

Methods, materials, validated information and training are all essential for tobacco control activities and require both financial and human resources. Compared with the resources deployed by the tobacco industry for the marketing of its products, the financial resources available for tobacco control are minute, hence the need to select carefully the tools to be used, preferably those that have several effects.

It has often proved difficult to find resources to implement tobacco control strategies, thus part of the role of the various strategists will be to mobilize resources or find alternative approaches. Such alternatives could include using censuses or other health surveys to gather the data required; twinning tobacco control programmes between countries with large resources and others with more meagre ones; forming coalitions and networking; using all those in positions of influence, from ministries to the media, for promotion and advocacy; and appropriating a certain percentage of tax revenue from tobacco products for health programmes aimed at women.

Political figures, especially women, in decision-making positions who have some interest in the subject are also an important resource, as are lobbyists for tobacco control.

Universities should be encouraged to undertake research and training on women and tobacco as part of their regular activities and to validate and publish information on women and tobacco.

Worldwide interest in tobacco control is leading to effective cooperation and alliance-building. Tobacco control among women

101

is greatly enhanced by the formation of coalitions and networks that permit communication and coordinated action. Coordination encourages sharing of information and strategies, permits efficient use of financial and personal resources, and eases the isolation often felt by individuals working in this area. Perhaps most importantly, these organizations greatly enhance the power of individuals to bring about changes.

Networks dedicated to the issue of women's use of tobacco are proliferating around the world. On an international level, the International Network of Women Against Tobacco (INWAT) was founded in 1990. INWAT's goals are to counter the targeted marketing and promotion of tobacco to women and girls, and to encourage the development of women-centred tobacco prevention and cessation programmes. INWAT's activities include the following:

— maintaining an international database of individuals working to address tobacco control among women;

— producing an international directory of women working in tobacco control;

— producing, collecting and distributing case-studies of efforts to undermine advertising targeted at women and of successful women-centred approaches to smoking prevention and cessation;

— ensuring that the issue of women and smoking has a more prominent place within the tobacco control movement.

Regional networks will also prove valuable, to allow members to focus on local issues and to develop the most appropriate strategies for particular areas. For example, the Association of Latin American Women for Smoking Control (AMALTA) was founded in 1991 to address tobacco use by women in Latin America.

Collecting funds or obtaining financial support for tobacco control has proved to be difficult enough in developed countries. Most developing countries are still struggling with communicable diseases and an acute lack of resources for primary health care. The responsibilities of the more developed countries in the implementation of the worldwide strategy for tobacco control among women need to be stressed. Their role in the transfer and adaptation of information on tobacco use among women and on measures to control it is fundamental; they are also often in a better economic position to participate in this transfer.

References

1. Wald N, Nicolaides-Bouman A. *UK smoking statistics*, 2nd ed. Oxford, Oxford University Press, 1991.

2. Weng XZ, Hong ZG, Chen DY. Smoking prevalence in Chinese aged 15 and above. *Chinese medical journal*, 1987, 100: 886-892.

3. Chapman S, Leng WW. *Tobacco control in the Third World. A resource atlas.* Penang, International Organization of Consumers' Unions, 1990.

4. Bartal M et al. Le tabagisme au Maroc, ébauche de lutte antitabac [An outline of Morocco's fight against tobacco use]. *Hygie*, 1988, 7: 30-32.

5. Tuomilehto J et al. Smoking rates in Pacific islands. *Bulletin of the World Health Organization*, 1986, 64: 447-456.

6. Pierce JM et al. Uptake and quitting smoking trends in Australia 1974-1984. *Preventive medicine*, 1987, 16: 252-260.

7. Fiore MC et al. Trends in cigarette smoking in the United States — the changing influence of gender and race. *Journal of the American Medical Association*, 1989, 261: 49-55.

8. Pierce JP et al. Trends in cigarette smoking — projections to the year 2000. *Journal of the American Medical Association*, 1989, 261: 61-65.

9. Health and Welfare Canada. *Canadians and smoking: an update*. Ottawa, Department of Health and Welfare, 1991.

10. Jacobson B. *Beating the ladykillers — women and smoking*. London, Victor Gollancz, 1988.

11. Rimpela M et al. *Changes in health habits of young people in Finland in 1977-1987*. Helsinki, Finnish National Board of Health, 1987 (Series original reports, No. 7).

12. Greaves L. *Background paper on women and tobacco*. Ottawa, Department of Health and Welfare, 1987.

13. *A new form of smokeless tobacco: moist snuff*. Report. Brussels, European Bureau for Action on Smoking Prevention, 1990.

14. Millar WJ. The use of chewing tobacco and snuff in Canada, 1986. *Canadian journal of public health*, 1989, 80: 131-135.

15. Haglund M. *Prevalence of smoking among teenage girls and women in Europe*. Paper presented to 2nd World No-Tobacco Day Conference, Copenhagen, WHO Regional Office for Europe, 1989.

16. Pierce JP et al. Trends in cigarette smoking in the United States — educational differences are increasing. *Journal of the American Medical Association*, 1989, 261: 56-60.

17. Action on Smoking and Health. *Women and smoking — a handbook for action*. London, Health Education Council, 1986.

103

18. *Taking control, an action handbook on women and tobacco.* Ottawa, Canadian Council on Smoking and Health, 1989.

19. Rosero-Bixby L, Oberle MW. Tobacco use in Costa Rican women. *Ciencias sociales,* 1987, 35: 95-102.

20. Elegbeleye OO, Femi-Pearse D. Incidence and variables contributing to onset of cigarette smoking among secondary school children and medical students in Lagos, Nigeria. *British journal of preventive and social medicine,* 1976, 30: 66-70.

21. Report from Ghana. In: *Smoking and health issues in selected English-speaking African countries. Report of a HQ/AFRO Regional Seminar on Smoking and Health, Lusaka, 26-28 June 1984.*

22. Swaziland National Council on Alcohol and Drug Dependence. Research project on smoking. In: *Smoking and health issues in selected English-speaking African countries. Report of a HQ/AFRO Regional Seminar on Smoking and Health, Lusaka, 26-28 June 1984.*

23. Haworth A, Mulenga M, Mwanza P. Report from Zambia. In: *Smoking and health issues in selected English-speaking African countries. Report of a HQ/AFRO Regional Seminar on Smoking and Health, Lusaka, 26-28 June 1984.*

24. Zein Ahmed Zein et al. Patterns of cigarette smoking among Ethiopian medical and paramedical students. *Ethiopian medical journal,* 1984, 22: 165-171.

25. Onadeko BO, Awotedie AA, Onadeko MO. Smoking patterns of students in higher institutions of learning in Nigeria. In: *Proceedings of the 5th World Conference on Smoking and Health, Winnipeg, 10-15 July 1983.* Ottawa, Canadian Council on Smoking and Health, 1983, p. 773.

26. Granworth H, Stanley K, Lopez AD. *Time trends in mortality for cancer.* WHO/CAN/88.5 (available on request from the Division of Noncommunicable Diseases and Health Technology, World Health Organization, 1211 Geneva 27, Switzerland).

27. Suhardi KDS et al. Dominant role of clove cigarette smoking patterns in Indonesia. In: Durston B, Jamrozik K, ed. *The global war. Abstracts of the 7th World Conference on Tobacco and Health, Perth, 1-5 April 1990.* Perth, Health Department of Western Australia, 1990, p. 241.

28. Aghi M, Gupta PC, Mehta FS. Impact of intervention on the reverse smoking habit of rural Indian women. In: Aoki M et al., ed. *Smoking and health. Proceedings of the 6th World Conference on Smoking and Health, Tokyo, 9-12 November 1987.* Amsterdam, Excerpta Medica, 1988, p. 255.

29. Said AK. Personal habits and health status. In: Fouad AE, Ibrahim AS, Mobarez AE, ed. *Health profile of Egypt. Report of the health interview survey. Second cycle. Part IV.* Ministry of Health, 1985 (Publication No. 32/4).

30. *The economic consequences of smoking in Egypt.* Cairo, Cairo University Cancer Institute, 1989.

31. Yason JV et al. Smoking among children in metropolitan Manila. *Phillipine journal of cardiology,* 1984, 12: 11-18.

32. Perdrizet S et al. Prévalence et étiologie des symptômes et affections respiratoires chez les adolescents scolarisés de Polynésie française [Prevalence and etiology of respiratory symptoms and affections in adolescent schoolchildren in French Polynesia]. *Revue française des maladies respiratoires,* 1982, 10: 143-149.

33. *The effects of active and passive smoking on the respiratory health of primary school children in Hong Kong.* Studies on respiratory health in Hong Kong, report 2. Hong Kong, University of Hong Kong, Department of Community Medicine and Paediatrics, 1991.

34. *The health consequences of smoking for women. A report of the Surgeon-General.* Rockville, MD, US Department of Health and Human Services, Public Health Service, Office on Smoking and Health, 1980.

35. Griner E. Life expectancies of cigarette smokers and non-smokers in the United States. *Social science and medicine*, 1991, 32: 1151-1159.

36. *Reducing the health consequences of smoking: 25 years of progress. A report of the Surgeon-General.* Rockville, MD, US Department of Health and Human Services, Public Health Service, Office on Smoking and Health, 1989 (DHHS Publication No. (CDC) 89-8411).

37. Stanley K et al. Women and cancer. *World health statistics quarterly*, 1987, 40: 267-278.

38. Koroltchouk V et al. Bladder cancer: approaches to prevention. *Bulletin of the World Health Organization*, 1987, 65: 513-520.

39. *The health consequences of involuntary smoking. A report of the Surgeon-General.* Rockville, MD, US Department of Health and Human Services, Public Health Service, Office on Smoking and Health, 1986 (DHHS Publication No. (CDC) 87-8398).

40. Feinleib M et al. Trends in COPD morbidity and mortality in the United States. *American review of respiratory disease*, 1989, 140: 509-518.

41. Davis RM, Novotny TE. Changes in risk factors. The epidemiology of cigarette smoking and its impact on chronic obstructive pulmonary disease. *American review of respiratory disease*, 1989, 140: 582-589.

42. Krishna K. Tobacco chewing in pregnancy. *British journal of obstetrics and gynaecology*, 1978, 85: 726-728.

43. Humble C et al. Passive smoking and 20-year cardiovascular disease mortality among non-smoking wives, Evans county, Georgia. *American journal of public health*, 1990, 80: 599-601.

44. Nakamura M et al. Effect of passive smoking during pregnancy on birth weight and gestation. In: Aoki M et al., ed. *Smoking and health. Proceedings of the 5th World Conference on Smoking and Health, Tokyo, 9-12 November 1987.* Amsterdam, Excerpta Medica, 1988, pp. 267-269.

45. Gortmalher SL et al. Parental smoking and the risk of childhood asthma. *American journal of public health*, 1982, 72: 575-579.

46. Cohen N. Smoking, health and survival: prospects in Bangladesh. *Lancet*, 1981, 1: 1090-1093.

47. *Not far enough: women vs smoking. A workshop for women's group and women's health leaders.* Rockville, MD, US Department of Health and Human Services, Public Health Service, Office on Smoking and Health, 1987.

48. Stanton WR et al. *The origins and development of an addictive behaviour: a longitudinal study of smoking. Summary and recommendations.* Dunedin, Dunedin Multidisciplinary Health and Development Research Unit, 1989.

49. Figa-Talamanca I, Modolo MA. Evaluation of an antismoking educational programme among adolescents in Italy. *Hygie*, 1989, 8: 24-28.

50. Nutbeam D et al. *Planning for a smoke-free generation.* Copenhagen, WHO Regional Office for Europe, 1988 (Smoke-free Europe series, No. 6).

51. Charlton A, Blair V. Predicting the onset of smoking in boys and girls. *Social science and medicine*, 1989, 29: 813-818.

52. Berg MA et al. *Health behaviour among Finnish adult population. Spring 1989.* Helsinki, National Public Health Institute, 1990 (Publication No. B1/1990).

105

53. Amos A, Jacobson B, White P. Cigarette advertising policy and coverage of smoking and health in British women's magazines. *Lancet*, 1991, 337: 93-96.

54. Pentz MA. The power of policy: the relationship of smoking policy to adolescent smoking. *American journal of public health*, 1989, 79: 357-362.

55. McNeill AD et al. Nicotine intake in young smokers: longitudinal study of saliva cotinine concentrations. *American journal of public health*, 1989, 79: 172-175.

56. McNeill AD. The development of dependence on smoking in children. *British journal of addiction*, 1991, 86: 589-592.

57. Graham H. The changing patterns of women's smoking. *Health visitor*, 1989, 62: 22-24.

58. *Teenage smoking. Research study conducted for health education authority.* London, MORI, 1990.

59. Altman DG et al. Reducing the illegal sale of cigarettes to minors. *Journal of the American Medical Association*, 1989, 261: 80-83.

60. *The health benefits of smoking cessation. A report of the Surgeon-General.* Rockville, MD, US Department of Health and Human Services, Public Health Service, Office on Smoking and Health, 1990 (DHSS Publication No. (CDC) 90-8416).

61. Greaves L. *The prevention and cessation of tobacco use: how are women a special case?* Paper presented at the 7th World Conference on Tobacco and Health, Perth, 1-5 April 1990.

62. Cummings KM et al. Physician advice to quit smoking: who gets it and who doesn't. *American journal of preventive medicine*, 1987, 3: 69-75.

63. Li VC et al. The effectiveness of smoking cessation advice given during routine medical care: physicians can make a difference. *American journal of preventive medicine*, 1987, 3: 81-86.

64. Larsson US et al. Patient-doctor communication on smoking and drinking: lifestyle in medical consultations. *Social science and medicine*, 1987, 25: 1129-1137.

65. Batlle E et al. Tobacco prevention in hospitals: long-term follow-up of a smoking control programme. *British journal of addiction*, 1991, 86: 709-717.

66. *Smoking and its effects on health. Report of a WHO Expert Committee.* Geneva, World Health Organization, 1975 (WHO Technical Report Series, No. 568).

67. *Controlling the smoking epidemic. Report of the WHO Expert Committee on Smoking Control.* Geneva, World Health Organization, 1979 (WHO Technical Report Series, No. 636).

68. *Smoking control strategies in developing countries. Report of a WHO Expert Committee.* Geneva, World Health Organization, 1983 (WHO Technical Report Series, No. 695).

69. *Smokeless tobacco control. Report of a WHO Study Group.* Geneva, World Health Organization, 1988 (WHO Technical Report Series, No. 773).

Selected further reading

In addition to the references given on pp. 103–106, the following sources of information may prove useful to readers. While some are of general interest, others are directly related to the subject matter of individual chapters.

General interest

Smoking and its effects on health. Report of a WHO Expert Committee. Geneva, World Health Organization, 1975 (WHO Technical Report Series, No. 568).

Controlling the smoking epidemic. Report of the WHO Expert Committee on Smoking Control. Geneva, World Health Organization, 1979 (WHO Technical Report Series, No. 636).

Smoking control strategies in developing countries. Report of a WHO Expert Committee. Geneva, World Health Organization, 1983 (WHO Technical Report Series, No. 695).

Smokeless tobacco control. Report of a WHO Study Group. Geneva, World Health Organization, 1988 (WHO Technical Report Series, No. 773).

Tobacco smoking. Lyon, International Agency for Research on Cancer, 1986 (IARC Monographs on the Evaluation of Carcinogenic Risks to Humans, No. 38).

Tobacco habits other than smoking; betel-quid and areca-nut chewing; and some related nitrosamines. Lyon, International Agency for Research on Cancer, 1985 (IARC Monographs on the Evaluation of Carcinogenic Risks to Humans, No. 37).

Peto R, Zaridge D, ed. *Tobacco: a major international health hazard.* Lyon, International Agency for Research on Cancer, 1986 (IARC Scientific Publications, No. 74).

In 1988, the WHO Regional Office for Europe prepared a series of booklets (Smoke-free Europe) for the first European Conference on Tobacco Policy.[1] The booklets, which were pub-

---

[1] Available on request from the WHO Regional Office for Europe, DK-2100 Copenhagen Ø, Denmark.

lished in English, French, German, Russian and Spanish, deal with the following areas of interest in the tobacco or health field:

— the physician's role;
— legislative strategies for a smoke-free Europe;
— the evaluation and monitoring of public action on tobacco;
— tobacco or health;
— helping smokers stop;
— planning for a smoke-free generation;
— why people smoked and why they are stopping;
— tobacco advertising and promotion;
— tobacco price and the smoking epidemic.

Since 1979, the US Department of Health and Human Services has issued regular reports by the Surgeon-General on smoking and health; the most relevant are:

The health consequences of smoking for women. A report of the Surgeon-General. Rockville, MD, US Department of Health and Human Services, Public Health Service, Office on Smoking and Health, 1980.

The health consequences of involuntary smoking. A report of the Surgeon-General. Rockville, MD, US Department of Health and Human Services, Public Health Service, Office on Smoking and Health, 1986 (DHSS Publication No. (CDC) 87-8398).

Reducing the health consequences of smoking: 25 years of progress. A report of the Surgeon-General. Rockville, MD, US Department of Health and Human Services, Public Health Service, Office on Smoking and Health, 1989 (DHSS Publication No. (CDC) 89-8411).

The health benefits of smoking cessation. A report of the Surgeon-General. Rockville, MD, US Department of Health and Human Services, Public Health Service, Office on Smoking and Health, 1990 (DHSS Publication No. (CDC) 90-8416).

Chapter 2

Aghi MB. Tobacco and the Indian woman. In: *Proceedings of the 5th World Conference on Smoking and Health, Winnipeg, 10-15 July 1983.* Ottawa, Canadian Council on Smoking and Health, 1983, p. 255.

Bachman JG et al. Racial/ethnic differences in smoking, drinking, and illicit drug use among American high school seniors, 1976-1989. *American journal of public health*, 1991, 81: 372-377.

Barry M. The influence of the US tobacco industry on the health, economy, and environment of developing countries. *New England journal of medicine*, 1991, 324: 917-920.

Haglund M. Development trends in smoking among women in Sweden — an analysis. In: Aoki M et al., ed. *Smoking and health. Proceedings of the 6th World Conference on Smoking and Health, Tokyo, 9-12 November 1987.* Amsterdam, Excerpta Medica, 1988, pp. 525-529.

Mackay J. *Smoking and women. Technical discussion.* Asian Consultancy on Tobacco Control. WHO Regional Office for the Western Pacific, Manila, 1989.

Masironi R, Rothwell K. Tendances et effets du tabagisme dans le monde [Smoking trends and effects worldwide]. *World health statistics quarterly*, 1988, 41: 228-241.

Nath UR. *Smoking: Third World alert.* Oxford, Oxford University Press, 1986.

Paine P, Gomes Pereire M. Are smoking behaviours different in industrialized and developing countries? *Hygie*, 1988, 7: 27-29.

Pirie PL et al. Smoking prevalence in a cohort of adolescents, including dropouts, and transfers. *American journal of public health*, 1988, 78: 176-178.

Rigatto M et al. Smoking control policies and female smoking habits in less developed countries. In: Rosenberg MJ, ed. *Smoking and reproductive health.* Littlehorn, Massachussetts, PSG Publishing, 1987, p. 207.

Waldron I et al. Gender differences in tobacco use in Africa, Asia, the Pacific and Latin America. *Social science and medicine*, 1988, 27: 1269-1275.

Whalen E. *A smoking gun: how the tobacco industry gets away with murder.* Philadelphia, USA, George F. Stickley, 1984.

Yach D. The impact of smoking in developing countries with special reference to Africa. *International journal of health services*, 1986, 16: 279-292.

Chapter 3

Aloia JF et al. Risk factors for postmenopausal osteoporosis. *American journal of medicine*, 1985, 78: 95-100.

American Academy of Pediatrics, Committee on Environmental Hazards. Involuntary smoking: a hazard to children. *Pediatrics*, 1986, 77: 755-757.

Baron JA, Greenberg ER. Cigarette smoking and estrogen-related disease in women. In: Rosenberg MJ, ed. *Smoking and reproductive health.* Littleton, Massachussetts, PSG Publishing, 1987, pp. 150-156.

Beiraghi SM et al. Effect of smokeless tobacco on plasma lipoproteins in adolescents. *Pediatric dentistry,* 1988, 10: 19-21.

Bonham GS, Wilson RW. Children's health in families with cigarette smokers. *American journal of public health*, 1981, 71: 290-293.

Boyle P. *Cigarette smoking and pancreas cancer risk.* Lyon, International Agency for Research on Cancer, 1990.

Charlton A. Children's coughs related to parental smoking. *British medical journal*, 1984, 288: 1647-1649.

Charlton A. Passive smoking and health risks to children: a review of the recent evidence. In: Aoki M et al., ed. *Smoking and health. Proceedings of the 6th World Conference on Smoking and Health, Tokyo, 9-12 November 1987.* Amsterdam, Excerpta Medica, 1988, pp. 271-274.

Chen Y et al. Influence of passive smoking on admissions for respiratory illness in early childhood. *British medical journal*, 1986, 293: 303-306.

Clarke EA, Morgan RW, Newman AM. Smoking as a risk factor in cancer of the cervix: additional evidence from a case-control study. *American journal of epidemiology*, 1982, 115: 59-66.

109

Cogswell JJ et al. Parental smoking, breast-feeding and respiratory infection in development of allergic diseases. *Archives of disease in childhood*, 1987, 62: 338-344.

Doll R, Peto R. The causes of cancer: quantitative estimates of avoidable risks of cancer in the United States today. *Journal of the National Cancer Institute*, 1981, 66: 1191-1308.

Fabrikant JI. Radon and lung cancer: the Beir IV report. *Health physics*, 1990, 59: 87-89.

Glantz S, Parmley W. Passive smoking and heart disease: epidemiology, physiology, and biochemistry. *Circulation*, 1991, 83: 1-12.

Greenberg RA et al. Ecology of passive smoking by young infants. *Journal of pediatrics*, 1989, 114: 774-780.

Gross F et al. *Management of arterial hypertension. A practical guide for the physician and allied health workers*. Geneva, World Health Organization, 1984.

Haglund B et al. Cigarette smoking as a risk factor for sudden infant death syndrome: a population-based study. *American journal of public health*, 1990, 80: 29-32.

Harlap S. Smoking and spontaneous abortion. In: Rosenberg MJ, ed. *Smoking and reproductive health*. Littleton, Massachussetts, PSG Publishing, 1987, p. 79.

Harlap S, Davies AM. Infant admissions to hospital and maternal smoking. *Lancet*, 1974, 1: 529-532.

Herrero R et al. Invasive cervical cancer and smoking in Latin America. *Journal of the National Cancer Institute*, 1989, 81: 205-211.

Higgins JE. Smoking and cancer: methodologic considerations. In: Rosenberg MJ, ed. *Smoking and reproductive health*. Littleton, Massachussetts, PSG Publishing, 1987, p. 193.

Holck SE et al. Lung cancer mortality and smoking habits: Mexican-American women. *American journal of public health*, 1982, 72: 38-42.

Janerich DT et al. Lung cancer and exposure to tobacco smoke in the household. *New England journal of medicine*, 1990, 323: 632-636.

Lam TH et al. Smoking, passive smoking and histological types in lung cancer in Hong Kong Chinese women. *British journal of cancer*, 1987, 56: 673-678.

La Vecchia C. Patterns of cigarette smoking and trends in lung cancer mortality in Italy. *Journal of epidemiology and community health*, 1985, 39: 157-164.

La Vecchia C et al. Cigarette smoking and the risk of cervical neoplasma. *American journal of epidemiology*, 1986, 123: 22-29.

Little RE, Peterson DR. Sudden infant death syndrome epidemiology: a review and update. *Epidemiologic reviews*, 1990, 12: 241-246.

Loewen GM, Romano CF. Lung cancer in women. *Journal of psychoactive drugs*, 1989, 21: 319-321.

Malloy MH et al. The association of maternal smoking with age and cause of infant death. *American journal of epidemiology*, 1988, 128: 46-55.

McConnochie KM, Roghmann KJ. Parental smoking, presence of older siblings, and family history of asthma increase risk of bronchitis. *American journal of diseases of children*, 1986, 140: 806-812.

Neuspiel DR et al. Parental smoking and post-infancy wheezing in children: a prospective chest study. *American journal of public health*, 1989, 79: 168-171.

O'Connor GT et al. The effect of passive smoking on pulmonary functions and nonspecific bronchial responsiveness in a population-based sample of children and young adults. *American review of respiratory disease*, 1987, 135: 800-804.

Palmer JR et al. "Low yield" cigarettes and the risk of nonfatal myocardial infarction in women. *New England journal of medicine*, 1989, 320: 1569-1573.

Pandey MR et al. *Chronic bronchitis and coronary pulmonale in Nepal*. Katmandu, Mrigendra Medical Trust, 1988.

Piper JM, Matanoski GM, Tonascia J. Bladder cancer in young women. *American journal of epidemiology*, 1986, 123: 1033-1042.

Pocock NA et al. Effects of tobacco use on axial and appendicular bone mineral density. *Bone*, 1991, 10: 95-100.

Riboli E et al. Exposure of nonsmoking women to environmental tobacco smoke: a 10-country collaborative study. *Cancer causes and control*, 1990, 1: 243-252.

Rosenberg L et al. Decline in the risk of myocardial infarction among women who stop smoking. *New England journal of medicine*, 1990, 322: 213-217.

Smith EM, Sowers MF, Burns TL. Effects of smoking on the development of female reproductive cancers. *Journal of the National Cancer Institute*, 1984, 73: 371-376.

Snider GL. Changes in COPD occurrence. Chronic obstructive pulmonary disease: a definition and implications of structural determinants of airflow obstruction for epidemiology. *American review of respiratory disease*, 1989, 140: 53-58.

Stergachis A et al. Maternal cigarette smoking and the risk of tubal pregnancy. *American journal of epidemiology*, 1991, 133: 332-337.

Tager IB. "Passive smoking" and respiratory health in children — sophistry or cause for concern? *American review of respiratory disease*, 1986, 133: 959-961.

Tager IB et al. Longitudinal study of the effects of maternal smoking on pulmonary function in children. *New England journal of medicine*, 1983, 309: 699-703.

Thom TJ. International comparisons in COPD mortality. *American review of respiratory disease*, 1989, 140: 527-534.

Trevathan E et al. Cigarette smoking and dysplasia and carcinoma *in situ* of the uterine cervix. *Journal of the American Medical Association*, 1983, 250: 499-502.

Weitzman M et al. Maternal smoking and childhood asthma. *Pediatrics*, 1990, 85: 505-509.

Winn DM et al. Snuff dipping and oral cancer among women in the southern United States. *New England journal of medicine*, 1981, 304: 745-749.

World Health Organization. Female lung cancer increases in developed countries. *Weekly epidemiological record*, 1986, 61: 297-299.

Wu AH et al. Smoking and other risk factors for lung cancer in women. *Journal of the National Cancer Institute*, 1985, 74: 747-751.

Chapter 4

Amos A, Bostock B. *Putting women in the picture: cigarette advertising policy and coverage of smoking and health in women's magazines in Europe*. London, British Medical Association, 1991.

Darbyshire P. Hiding behind the smokescreen. *Nursing times*, 1986, 16: 48-50.

Davis RM. Current trends in cigarette advertising and marketing. *New England journal of medicine*, 1987, 316: 725-732.

Ernster VL. Mixed messages for women: a social history of cigarette smoking and advertising. *New York state journal of medicine*, 1985, 316: 725-732.

Facts and reflections on girls and substance use. New York, Girls Inc., 1989.

Goddard F, Ikin L. *Smoking among secondary school children.* London, HMSO, 1986.

Grunberg NE, Winders SE, Wewers ME. Gender differences in tobacco use. *Health psychology*, 1991, 10: 143-153.

Haines J. Women: targets of a tobacco industry pressure. *Canadian nurse*, 1988, 84: 15-17.

Hogue CJR, Berman SM. Smoking and the women's movement. In: Rosenberg MJ, ed. *Smoking and reproductive health.* Littleton, Massachussetts, PSG Publishing, 1987, pp. 23-25.

A manual on smoking and children. Geneva, International Union against Cancer, 1982 (UICC Technical Report Series, No. 73).

Michell L. *Growing up in smoke.* London, Pluto Press, 1990.

Pandey MR, Neupane RP, Gautam A. Epidemiological study of tobacco smoking behaviour among adults in a rural community of the Hill region of Nepal with special reference to attitude and beliefs. *International journal of epidemiology*, 1988, 17: 535-541.

Piepe T et al. Girls smoking and self-esteem — the adolescent context. *Health education journal*, 1988, 47: 83-85.

Pirie PL et al. Gender differences in cigarette smoking and quitting in a cohort of young adults. *American journal of public health*, 1991, 81: 324-327.

Smith GD, Shipley MJ. Confounding of occupation and smoking: its magnitude and consequences. *Social science and medicine*, 1991, 32: 1297-1300.

Steinem G. Sex, lies and advertising. *Ms. magazine*, 1990, July/August.

Waldron I. Patterns and causes of gender differences in smoking. *Social science and medicine*, 1991, 32: 989-1005.

Warner K. *Selling smoke: cigarette advertising and public health.* Washington, DC, American Public Health Association, 1986.

Warner KE. Cigarette advertising and media coverage of smoking and health. *New England journal of medicine*, 1985, 312: 384-388.

Chapter 5

Bellew B, Wayne D. Prevention of smoking among school children: a review of research and recommendations. *Health education journal*, 1991, 50: 3-8.

Bultz B et al. Successful smoking cessation. *Canadian nurse*, 1988, 19: 18-20.

Catching our breath. A journal about change for women who smoke. Winnipeg, Manitoba, Women's health clinic, 1990.

Delaney SF. *Women smokers can quit: a different approach.* Evanston, IL, Women's Healthcare Press, 1989.

Flay BR. *Selling the smokeless society: fifty-six evaluated mass media programs and campaigns worldwide.* Washington, DC, 1987 (American public health practice series).

Frankowski BL et al. Advising parents to stop smoking. Opportunities and barriers in pediatric care. *American journal of diseases of children,* 1989, 143: 1091-1094.

Frese PA, Schierling-Wilkes J. Smokeless tobacco. The role of the dental hygienist. *Dental hygiene,* 1987: 366-369.

Graham H. Women and smoking in the UK: the implications for health promotion. *Health promotion,* 1989, 3: 371-382.

Johansson G, Johnson J, Hall E. Smoking and sedentary behaviour as related to work organization. *Social science and medicine,* 1991, 32: 837-846.

Kretzschmar RM. Smoking and health: the role of the obstetrician and gynecologist. *Obstetrics and gynecology,* 1980, 55: 403-406.

Mosbach P, Leventhal H. Peer group identification and implications for intervention. *Journal of abnormal psychology,* 1988, 97: 238-245.

Noppa H, Bengtsson C. Obesity in relation to smoking: a population study of women in Goteborg, Sweden. *Preventive medicine,* 1980, 9: 534-543.

Pekurinen M, Valtonen H. Price, policy and consumption of tobacco: the Finnish experience. *Social science and medicine,* 1987, 25: 875-881.

Perkins KA et al. The effect of nicotine on energy expenditure during light physical activity. *New England journal of medicine,* 1989, 320: 898-903.

Prochaska JO, Di Clemente OC. States and processes of self-change of smoking. *Journal of consulting and clinical psychology,* 1983, 51: 390-395.

Rigotti NA. Cigarette smoking and weight gain. *New England journal of medicine,* 1989, 320: 931-933.

Schwartz J. *Review and evaluation of smoking cessation and methods: the United States and Canada, 1978-1985.* Washington, DC, US Department of Health and Human Services, 1987.

The smoking digest: progress report and a nation kicking the habit. Washington, DC, US Department of Health and Human Services, 1977.

Stewart A, Orme J. Teenage smoking and health education. *Health visitor,* 1989, 62: 91-94.

Sullivan LW. Protect young people from tobacco addiction. *State health legislation report,* 1990.

Williamson DF et al. Smoking cessation and severity of weight gain in a national cohort. *New England journal of medicine,* 1991, 324: 739-745.

Chapter 6

Leppo K, Vertio H. Smoking control in Finland: a case study in policy formulation and implementation. *Health promotion,* 1986, 1: 5-16.

McLellan DL. *Toward an international network of women against tobacco.* Paper presented at "Women, tobacco, and health" workshop, 7th World Conference on Tobacco and Health, Perth, 30 March 1990.

Roemer R. *Legislative action to combat the world tobacco epidemic,* 2nd ed. Geneva, World Health Organization, in press.

Annex 1

Survey on tobacco use

The following format has been designed for the systematic collection of information on national tobacco control programmes. It comprises a set of questions for the establishment of a country profile and a set of definitions and notes to assist countries to complete the questionnaire.

Through the use of a standard format, WHO is trying to ensure worldwide compatibility of data. However, it is realized that the availability of information on tobacco use will vary considerably in different countries and hence some degree of flexibility is anticipated. Some countries may have additional information; in other countries, a lack of information regarding some of the questions should not prevent their completing other items of the profile for which information is available.

The name and functions of the persons responsible for collecting the information and for updating it should be mentioned, together with the dates on which the profile or individual data therein was updated.

Summary country profile

1. Tobacco consumption, prevalence and intensity

1.1 Total national consumption in kg:

	1990	1989	1988	1987	1986	1985
All tobacco products combined						
Cigarettes						
Cigars and pipe tobacco						
Other forms (e.g. bidi, hookah and chewing tobacco)						

115

1.2 Are periodic surveys or other assessments conducted of cigarette/tobacco consumption and of smoking prevalence and intensity according to sex, age group and specific population subgroups? (e.g. occupation, urban/rural residence, socio-economic status, geographical subdivisions.)

1.3 If so, for which year(s) during the past decade or so are the data available?

1.4 Are other forms of tobacco use also included in these surveys? If so, please provide details.

1.5 Smoking prevalence and intensity:

	Period 1			Period 2		
	Males	Females	Date	Males	Females	Date
1. Percentage of population aged 15 years and over who are regular smokers						
2. Percentage of population who are regular smokers, by age group: — 10–14 years — 15–19 years — 20–24 years — 25–44 years — 45–64 years — 65 years and over						
3. Smoking prevalence (%) in specific population subgroups (e.g. by occupation, race, ethnicity, socio-economic status, education)						
4. Among regular tobacco users, average consumption per day of: — cigarettes — cigars or pipe tobacco — other tobacco products						
5. Percentage of population who are ex-smokers						

1.6 Please provide the information requested below for the major brands of cigarettes (maximum of 5) sold in your country, together with their respective market shares (if known).

116

Brand and type (menthol, filter, etc.)	Tar (mg per cigarette)	Nicotine (mg per cigarette)	Filter tip (Yes or No)	Market share (%)	Year
a.	....	....	....	....	....
b.	....	....	....	....	....
c.	....	....	....	....	....
d.	....	....	....	....	....
e.	....	....	....	....	....

1.7   Is there any information on the average age at which people begin smoking in your country? If so, what is the proportion of adult smokers who report beginning to smoke during the following ages? (Please provide data for the latest period available.)

Age	Men (%)	Women (%)	Both (%)	Year of survey
10 years and under	....	....	....	....
11–14 years	....	....	....	....
15–19 years	....	....	....	....
20 years and over	....	....	....	....
Mean age	....	....	....	....

2.   Mortality and morbidity from tobacco-related diseases

2.1   Mortality rate or number of deaths from various causes:

	Period 1			Period 2		
	Males	Females	Date	Males	Females	Date
Total deaths						
Lung cancer						
Cancer of the larynx						
Cancer of the lip, oral cavity and pharynx						
Other cancers						
Bronchitis and emphysema						
Cardiovascular diseases (stroke, myocardial infarction)						
Acute upper respiratory infections						
All causes						

117

2.2 Is there high mortality from any other disease which may be associated, partly with smoking and partly with another traditional use of tobacco or endemic disease in your country? (e.g. bladder cancer — schistosomiasis and smoking — or oesophageal cancer — use of alcohol and smoking.) If so, please provide mortality data for the two periods shown in the table above.

2.3 Does your country use these data to regularly assess the mortality attributable to tobacco use? (or smoking?)

2.4 If so, how is your country monitoring the number of deaths attributable to tobacco use? (or smoking?)

2.5 Number of deaths attributable to tobacco use:

	Period 1			Period 2		
	Males	Females	Date	Males	Females	Date
Total						
Lung cancer						
Cancer of the larynx						
Cancer of the lip, oral cavity and pharynx						
Other cancers						
Bronchitis and emphysema						
Cardiovascular diseases						

2.6 Does your country monitor the amount of morbidity caused by tobacco use?

2.7 If so, please provide whatever information is available for the two data periods shown above. These data may be national or regional or refer to a specific locality, e.g. a hospital catchment area. Where possible, information should be shown separately for inpatients and outpatients and for the major tobacco-related diseases.

2.8 Does your country monitor the health care costs and economic losses (e.g. caused by absenteeism) due to tobacco use?

2.9 If so, please provide any available information for the two data periods shown above.

3. Economics and tobacco

3.1 Please provide comparative figures or estimates for your country for each of the past 10 years (or for the longest and most recent period available) on the following:

— annual tobacco production, import and export;

— annual cigarette production, import and export;

— annual production of other manufactured tobacco goods, import and export.

3.2 Please provide comparative figures or estimates for each of the past 10 years on the annual income/expenses (in local currency) from tobacco production and consumption in your country through:

— monetary value of agricultural production of tobacco;

— monetary value of the manufacture of tobacco products;

— cost of imports of tobacco, cigarettes and other manufactured tobacco products;

— revenue raised by taxation (customs and excise taxes) on tobacco products as a percentage of all taxes;

— income from tobacco exports.

3.3 How is the revenue from tobacco used? Is any part of this revenue used for health-care services, health promotion campaigns, and/or social expenses?

3.4 How many jobs are generated annually as a result of tobacco production and distribution? (Number of people employed in the production, manufacturing and distribution sectors of the tobacco industry.)

3.5 Have any alternative crops been tried? If so, please provide details of the programme and outcome.

3.6 What is the cost of 20 cigarettes and the mean household income per year?

4. Health education

4.1 What are the components of the anti-tobacco health education programmes for schoolchildren in your country? At what age is anti-tobacco education introduced? What form does this school education take? Is it integrated into a global health education curriculum? Has it been evaluated?

4.2 How is health education on the dangers of tobacco presented in the curricula of health personnel such as doctors and specialists, nurses, dentists, dental hygienists, dieticians and others?

4.3 Are public information programmes (anti-smoking messages) organized systematically or for special occasions (e.g. World No-Tobacco Day) on the following media: television, radio, press, others? Please give examples. How often are they featured?

4.4 Are community anti-smoking activities, including smoking cessation programmes, organized? If so, at what level and for which specific groups? (e.g. women, pregnant women, migrant workers.) Please give examples. How are health personnel involved?

4.5 What is the role of governmental and nongovernmental organizations, respectively, in health education?

4.6 What is the government budget for health education?

4.7 What proportion of this budget is allocated to anti-smoking health education programmes?

5. Legislation and regulation

5.1 What are the laws or regulations that have been adopted in your country to restrict smoking in public places such as public transport, official buildings, schools, etc.? How are these restrictions enforced? In what year did these laws or regulations come into force?

5.2 What are the laws protecting children from tobacco?
   • Which laws prohibit the sale of tobacco products to minors?
   • Is there is a ban on tobacco-vending machines in your country?
   • Is smoking prohibited in schools or other educational institutions?

5.3 Is smoking prohibited in health and health-related premises such as hospitals (public or private), health centres, screening facilities, ambulances, doctors' offices, dental surgeries, etc.? When did these regulations come into force?

5.4 Is there a ban (direct or indirect) on the advertising of tobacco products? Please provide details. To which form of media does this ban apply?

5.5 Is there a ban on the sponsorship of sporting or cultural events by tobacco companies? How is this ban enforced?

5.6 What are the regulations on the labelling of tobacco/cigarette packets?
  - What are the health warnings marked on tobacco packets? Are these health warnings changed regularly? What is the size of these warnings compared with the size of the tobacco packet?
  - Is it compulsory to indicate tar and nicotine yields on tobacco packets?
  - Is it compulsory to list the additives to the tobacco on the packets?

5.7 Has any other legislative action been taken in your country against tobacco? Are these laws enforced? If so, by whom?

6. Behavioural, cultural and sociological factors

6.1 Have any studies been conducted on the sociological and cultural determinants of smoking in the general population or in specific groups, e.g. young people, women, and minority groups? (Please give details.)

6.2 How is public knowledge about the effects of tobacco use surveyed? How often is it surveyed? What percentage of the population consider smoking to be harmful?

6.3 How is social acceptability of tobacco use evaluated in your country? How often is it evaluated? Is it decreasing?

6.4 What is the general attitude of the public to tobacco regulations? Is it surveyed?

7. General policy and programme matters

7.1 Is there a national focal point, such as a national organization or group of health agencies formally in charge of the tobacco control activities or the coordination of these activities? How is it funded? In which structure (governmental or otherwise) is it located? How many paid staff does it have? Please give address, phone number, etc. of the organizations involved.

7.2 Are there any nongovernmental organizations or special groups addressing the "tobacco or health" issue?

7.3 Does your government have an official policy or programme addressing all (or most) of the above-mentioned points (1.1–6.4)? If so, please provide details and attach relevant documentation. What proportion of total government expenditure is allocated to the implementation of this policy/programme?

121

7.4 Have the anti-tobacco measures taken in your country been effective? Please explain how they have been enforced. What results have been obtained?

7.5 Can you give any other information on the effectiveness of the tobacco control policy/strategy/programme being implemented at present in your country?

8.   Other related information

For example, future plans, areas of specific interest, etc.

Guidance for the completion of the country profile

1.   Tobacco consumption, prevalence and intensity

This section of the questionnaire is concerned with statistical information on tobacco use and tobacco-related disease in your country. Information should be provided on any form of tobacco consumption which you consider to have significant consequences for the health of the population.

The definitions and data format pertaining to this section are those adopted by WHO for collecting information at the international level on tobacco consumption and related diseases. It would be helpful if the data could be provided according to the definitions and format specified; however, any information that is available on these topics would greatly assist WHO in monitoring the tobacco epidemic. If the format and definitions differ from those suggested here, please specify the definitions, ages, population groups, etc. which are relevant for your country in order to assist WHO in interpreting the data.

Question 1.1

This question refers to the annual national consumption of tobacco products (in kg if possible). These estimates are generally derived from trade balance sheets, taking into account data on imports, exports, production and stockpiling of tobacco products. If available, consumption data should be provided according to the major forms of tobacco use as indicated and for as many years as possible.

Data on the prevalence of use of the various tobacco products should also be provided if possible.

122

Questions 1.2–1.5

Smoking prevalence is usually defined as the percentage of a particular population being surveyed who are regular smokers (see question 1.5, Item 1, below, for a definition of regular smokers). For monitoring purposes it is extremely important that prevalence be assessed within specific population subgroups, and in particular by age and sex (see Question 1.5). In addition, prevalence should also be assessed by demographic characteristics such as occupation (or some other indicator of socioeconomic status) and place of residence.

Surveys may be national surveys of prevalence or they may be less comprehensive (e.g. urban residents or certain localities) with known sampling biases (e.g. poorer segments of the population may have been excluded). The nature of the survey should be specified. If possible, nationally representative survey data should be reported.

Survey or census data on prevalence of tobacco use may refer to a single calendar year or several years. It should be specified when the data were collected. If prevalence data are not available for the 1980s, information for the latest year(s) available should be provided.

Question 1.5

The purpose of this table is to provide information on tobacco use, now and at some earlier period. Ideally, the two periods should be about 10 years apart, although you may wish to provide data for a shorter or longer period, depending on availability and relevance to the assessment of programme effectiveness.

Period 1 should be used for the latest available data. The data need not necessarily be confined to a single calendar year, but may include 2, 3 or even 5 years. Furthermore, the data for each item under Period 1 may not be available for the same calendar year(s). For example, data on regular smokers aged 15 and over may be available for 1990, but detailed age-specific data may only be available for 1988. In this case, please specify the reference year(s) for each item in the column provided.

Period 2 should be used for data referring to a period about 10 years earlier than Period 1. Data should be shown for as many items as possible, even if the calendar year(s) are not the same for each item. Please specify the reference year(s) where necessary.

Item 1. A *regular smoker* is someone who, at the time of the survey, smokes some kind of tobacco product every day and has done so for the last 6 months or more. A comparable definition may be used for other forms of tobacco use (e.g. chewing

123

tobacco). The definition does not include *occasional smokers* (i.e. anyone who smokes, but less than once a day). However, if your definition of regular smoker includes occasional smokers, please indicate this on the questionnaire.

If prevalence data are not available for the population aged 15 years and over, please provide any data that are available and indicate accordingly.

Item 2. If prevalence data are not available for the age groups indicated, please provide data for whatever age groups are available.

Item 3. Prevalence data may be available for certain population subgroups, according to occupation, socioeconomic status (however defined), urban/rural residence, administrative divisions (e.g. states/provinces), etc. A maximum of five subgroups should be selected.

Item 4. For those who are reported to be regular tobacco users, data is required on their average daily consumption of tobacco products, including:

— manufactured cigarettes;
— hand-rolled cigarettes;
— bidis;
— pipefuls of tobacco;
— cigars;
— pinches of snuff;
— quids of chewing tobacco, etc.

If consumption data are not available in this format, please provide them in whatever format is available.

2. Mortality and morbidity from tobacco-related diseases

In view of the rising incidence of tobacco-related diseases in many countries, various techniques have been developed for assessing the annual rates of mortality and/or morbidity due to tobacco use, particularly smoking.

Question 2.5

The table requests data on the total number of deaths attributable to tobacco use over all ages. If data are available by age group, and/or for specific forms of tobacco use (e.g. cigarettes), please provide them. As for Question 1.5, the two periods may each comprise one or more calendar years, and should be approximately one decade apart.

The table also requests information on the annual number of tobacco-attributable deaths coded to the major tobacco-related diseases, e.g. lung cancer. If desired, more specific categories may be reported. Thus "other cancers" may be further subdivided into oral cancer and/or oesophageal cancer and/or laryngeal cancer, all of which are significantly associated with tobacco use. The term "cardiovascular diseases" covers all diseases of the circulatory system, although more specific diseases, e.g. ischaemic heart disease, may be identified if data are available. Chronic obstructive lung diseases refer primarily to chronic bronchitis and emphysema.

Question 2.6

Please specify how the mortality or morbidity attributable to tobacco use is assessed. (Techniques range from applying fixed proportions calculated from studies in other countries (e.g. 90% for lung cancer, 75% for chronic obstructive lung disease and 25% for cardiovascular disease) to the use of findings from national studies on relative risks for smokers, in combination with detailed prevalence data for the population.)

Question 2.8

A number of countries have been monitoring the cost of the tobacco epidemic including direct costs of medical care (e.g. duration of stay in hospital, costs of treatment and costs of admission) and economic losses arising from lost productivity (e.g. absenteeism from work). Please provide whatever data are available, for the latest available year(s), and for some period about 10 years earlier.

3. Economics and tobacco

This section deals with the revenue accrued through tobacco production, processing and taxation; or alternatively with the expenses incurred through tobacco imports for non-tobacco producing countries. If specific surveys have been conducted, please attach the results.

Questions 3.1 and 3.2

The answers to these questions should provide an economic profile of the tobacco or health situation in individual countries, based on:

— revenue from production and manufacturing of tobacco products;

125

— cost of imports (to assess the impact of tobacco imports on the balance of trade);

— revenue from taxation (to analyse the income for the government from customs and excise taxes);

— income from exports (to assess the impact of tobacco exports on the balance of trade).

Question 3.3

How is the income generated by the production, manufacturing and distribution of tobacco used? Is the revenue put to a specific use? Please provide details. Can the income generated by tobacco be linked to health and social development in the country?

Question 3.5

The answer to this question should mention any attempt, general or partial, made to replace tobacco by other crops (e.g. groundnuts, maize, fruits or vegetables). The results of these experiences should be evaluated in relation to the financial outcome for the grower and for the state (if applicable).

4. Health education

Please attach the text of relevant courses or curricula.

Question 4.2

Please include training and postgraduate training as well as "on-the-job" retraining.

Question 4.3

Some people are still not aware of the damage to their health caused by smoking and other uses of tobacco. The facts, along with recent findings, should be publicized through an information programme. In order to reach the widest public, all those involved in the health field should participate in the programme and all forms of the media should be used.

Question 4.5

Please include the names of any nongovernmental organizations that play a role in anti-tobacco education.

5. Legislation

Please attach the text of the laws relevant to tobacco control.

Questions 5.1–5.3

The purpose of this section is to establish how much protection is given to the population against involuntary exposure to tobacco smoke. These measures may be valid nationally (legislation) or be the responsibility of local authorities (regulations).

Question 5.1

If the legislation provides for certain persons or communities to decide where smoking is permitted, it will be necessary to mention the main legislation and if possible to give an idea of the total impact of this legislation on smoke-free public places. If fines can be applied, please give details.

6. Behavioural, cultural and sociological factors

Surveys of public knowledge about tobacco could include questions on the harmful health consequences of tobacco use, the benefits of cessation, the hazards of passive smoking, etc. Public awareness may be assessed formally through national surveys or through more modest enquiries conducted at such places as the workplace. The nature of the survey should be specified.

7. General policy and programme matters

The issues mentioned in the six previous sections are often grouped in a tobacco control policy or programme. Many organizations and groups may play a role in the implementation of this policy or programme, the goal of which is a tobacco-free society. This set of questions is designed to determine the extent (and success) of the national policy and the organizations and groups involved.

Question 7.1

National focal points are usually located in the Ministry of Health, but in some cases a nongovernmental organization may be in charge of the coordination of and support for tobacco control activities.

127

Questions 7.4 and 7.5

These questions attempt to evaluate the effectiveness and completeness of national control programmes. Any information that is available on this subject should be given, even if it does not fall directly within the framework of the questions.